# Drug Speller
# 2009

# Drug Speller 2009

Dictionary Jumpstart, Inc.

# Drug Speller
# 2009

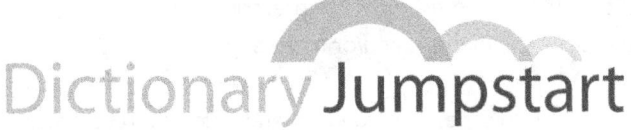

## Copyright © 2009 by Dictionary Jumpstart, Inc.

## NOTICE

Many of the drugs and/or products listed in this publication are protected by copyright, trademark or patent law and such designations are omitted for ease of use in this publication.

## TYPOGRAPHY

Various drug and medical product manufacturers prefer specific typographical characterizations of their products such as the mixing of upper and lower case letters and the insertion of hyphens, et cetera... Where possible, these preferences have been followed. However, these proprietary preferences are often disregarded in medical literature. Therefore, this book has chosen to use the most common typographical representations of drugs and/or products.

While every effort has been made to assure the accuracy of the spellings and categorizations contained in this publication, errors can occur and the author is not liable for any damages arising from the use or misuse of this publication. Furthermore, drugs are commonly used in multiple medical specialities for diverse reasons. The author's categorization of drugs is based upon the more common use of the drugs so categorized.

## RECOMMENDED USE OF THIS BOOK

This publication is designed to be used only by skilled professionals in researching the spelling of terminology. It should not be used for the prescribing or the taking of medication or in determining the proper use of drugs and/or medical products.

Nothing in this book should be construed as endorsing or recommending any drug or medical product.

Copies of this book can be purchased online at **www.drugspeller.com**

## A

- abacavir
- abatacept
- Abbokinase
- Abbo-Pac
- abciximab
- Abelcet
- Abilify
- Abilify Discmelt
- Abraxane
- Abreva
- Absorbine Jr
- ABX-EGF
- AC2993
- ACAM2000
- acamprosate
- Acanya
- acarbose
- acebutolol
- Accolate
- Accretropin
- Accuneb
- Accupril
- Accurbron
- Accuretic
- Accutane
- Accuzyme
- acebutolol
- ACE inhibitors
- Acel-Imune
- Aceon
- Acephen
- ACES
- Acetadote
- acetaminophen
- Acetasol
- acetazolamide
- acetohexamide
- acetohydroxamic acid
- acetyl sulfisoxazole
- acetylcysteine
- acetylsalicylic acid

## A

- Achromycin
- acid mantle creme
- acid phosphatase
- Aci-Jel
- AcipHex
- Acitretin
- Aclasta
- Aclovate
- Acomplia
- Acova
- Acrivastine
- ACTH
- Acthar
- Acthrel
- ActHIB
- Actical
- Acticin
- Actidel
- Actidose
- Actidose-Aqua
- Actifed
- Actigall
- Actimmune
- Actin
- Actiq
- ACTIS
- Activa Dystonia Therapy
- Activase
- Activella
- Activelle
- Actiza
- Actonel
- ACTOplus met
- Actos
- Acular
- Acuneb
- Acuprin 81
- AcuTect
- Acutrim
- acyclovir
- acycloguanosine

| A | A |
|---|---|

- ❏ Aczone
- ❏ Adacel
- ❏ Adagen
- ❏ Adalat
- ❏ Adalimumab
- ❏ Adamet
- ❏ adapalene
- ❏ Adderall
- ❏ Adeflor M
- ❏ Adefovir dipivoxil
- ❏ Adenocard
- ❏ Adenoscan
- ❏ adenosine
- ❏ Adipex
- ❏ Adipex-P
- ❏ Adoxa
- ❏ adrenocorticoids
- ❏ AdreView
- ❏ Adriamycin
- ❏ Adrucil
- ❏ Adsorbocarpine
- ❏ Advair Diskus
- ❏ Advair HFA
- ❏ Advate
- ❏ Advicor
- ❏ Advil
- ❏ Advil Liqui-Gels
- ❏ AeroBid
- ❏ AeroChamber
- ❏ AeroCount
- ❏ Aerolate
- ❏ Aerolone
- ❏ Aerophylline
- ❏ Aeroseb-DX
- ❏ Aerosporin
- ❏ Afeditab CR
- ❏ Affinitak
- ❏ Aflaxen
- ❏ Aflexa
- ❏ Aftate
- ❏ Afluria

- ❏ Afrin
- ❏ Aftate
- ❏ Agalsidase
- ❏ Agenerase
- ❏ aggrastat
- ❏ Aggrenox
- ❏ Agoral
- ❏ Agrylin
- ❏ AHA
- ❏ AH-Chew
- ❏ AHF
- ❏ A-hydroCort
- ❏ AidsVax
- ❏ Airet
- ❏ AK-Chlor
- ❏ AK-Con
- ❏ AK-Dilate
- ❏ AK-Fluor
- ❏ Akne-Mycin
- ❏ AK-Nefrin
- ❏ Akineton
- ❏ Akorn antioxidants
- ❏ AK-Pentolate
- ❏ AK-Poly
- ❏ AK-Pred
- ❏ Akpro
- ❏ Akrinol
- ❏ AK-Rinse
- ❏ AK-Spore
- ❏ AK-Sulf
- ❏ Akten
- ❏ Aktob
- ❏ AK-Tracin
- ❏ AK-Trol
- ❏ Akwa Tears
- ❏ ALA
- ❏ Alacol DM Syrup
- ❏ Alamast
- ❏ alatrofloxacin
- ❏ Alavert
- ❏ Alaway

## A

- ❑ Albalon
- ❑ Albamycin
- ❑ Albatussin SR
- ❑ albendazole
- ❑ Albenza
- ❑ albuferon
- ❑ Albumarc
- ❑ albumin
- ❑ Albuminar
- ❑ Albutein
- ❑ albuterol
- ❑ albuterol sulfate
- ❑ Alcaine
- ❑ alclometasone
- ❑ Alcomicin
- ❑ Alconefrin 12
- ❑ Aldactazide
- ❑ Aldactone
- ❑ Aldara
- ❑ aldesleukin
- ❑ Aldoclor
- ❑ Aldomet
- ❑ Aldoril
- ❑ Aldurazyme
- ❑ Alefacept
- ❑ Alemtuzumab
- ❑ alendronate
- ❑ Aleve
- ❑ Alfenta
- ❑ Alfentanil
- ❑ Alferon N
- ❑ alfuzosin
- ❑ Agalsidase beta
- ❑ Alglucerase
- ❑ alglucosidase alfa
- ❑ Align
- ❑ Alimentum Protein
- ❑ Alimta
- ❑ Alinia
- ❑ aliskiren
- ❑ AlitraQ Nutrition

## A

- ❑ Alitretinoin
- ❑ alkaline phosphatase
- ❑ Alka-Mints
- ❑ Alka-Seltzer
- ❑ Alkeran
- ❑ Allantoin
- ❑ All-Basic
- ❑ Allegra
- ❑ Allegra-D
- ❑ Allergan Lacri-Lube
- ❑ AllerNaze
- ❑ AlleRx
- ❑ Allfen
- ❑ Alli
- ❑ allium cepa
- ❑ allobarbital
- ❑ allopurinol
- ❑ Almotriptan malate
- ❑ Alocril
- ❑ aloe vera
- ❑ Alomide
- ❑ Alophen
- ❑ Aloprim
- ❑ Alora
- ❑ alosetron
- ❑ Aloxi
- ❑ alpha adrenergic receptor blockers
- ❑ alpha chymotrypsin
- ❑ Alpha Keri
- ❑ Alpha Lipoic
- ❑ Alpha Tocopherol
- ❑ Alpha-Hydroxy
- ❑ alpha-linolenic acid
- ❑ Alpha-Proteinase
- ❑ Alphagan
- ❑ Alphanate
- ❑ AlphaNine
- ❑ Alphatrex
- ❑ alprazolam
- ❑ alprostadil
- ❑ Alrex

| A | A |
|---|---|
| ❑ Altabax | ❑ Amigen |
| ❑ Altace | ❑ Amikacin |
| ❑ alteplase | ❑ Amikin |
| ❑ Alternagel | ❑ amiloride |
| ❑ Altinac | ❑ amino acid |
| ❑ Altocor | ❑ aminobenzoate |
| ❑ Altoprev | ❑ aminocaproic acid |
| ❑ Altramucil | ❑ Amino-Cerv |
| ❑ altretamine | ❑ aminoglutethimide |
| ❑ Alu-Cap | ❑ aminoglycoside |
| ❑ Aludrox | ❑ aminohippurate |
| ❑ Alumadrine | ❑ Aminolete |
| ❑ aluminum acetate | ❑ aminolevulinic acid |
| ❑ aluminum hydroxide | ❑ Aminomine |
| ❑ Alupent | ❑ aminophylline |
| ❑ Alustra | ❑ Aminoplex |
| ❑ Alvesco | ❑ aminosalicylic acid |
| ❑ alvimopan | ❑ Aminostasis |
| ❑ amantadine | ❑ Aminosyn |
| ❑ Amaryl | ❑ Aminotate |
| ❑ Ambenyl | ❑ Aminovirox |
| ❑ Ambien | ❑ Aminoxin |
| ❑ Ambifed | ❑ amiodarone |
| ❑ AmBisome | ❑ amithiozone |
| ❑ ambrisentan | ❑ Amitiza |
| ❑ amcinonide | ❑ Amitone |
| ❑ Amdoxovir | ❑ amitriptyline |
| ❑ Amen | ❑ AmLactin AP |
| ❑ Amerge | ❑ AmLactin XL |
| ❑ Americaine | ❑ amlexanox |
| ❑ Amerifed | ❑ amlodipine |
| ❑ Amerituss AD | ❑ amlodipine besylate |
| ❑ Amertan | ❑ ammonium chloride |
| ❑ AmethaPred | ❑ ammonium lactate |
| ❑ Amethopterin | ❑ Ammonul |
| ❑ Amevive | ❑ Amnesteem |
| ❑ Amfedsul | ❑ Amnestrogen |
| ❑ AMG 073 | ❑ amobarbital |
| ❑ Amicar | ❑ Amox Clav Pot |
| ❑ Amidate | ❑ amoxapine |
| ❑ amifostine | ❑ amoxicillin |

| A | A |
|---|---|
| ❏ Amoxil | ❏ Android |
| ❏ ampakine | ❏ Andropository injection |
| ❏ Amphadase | ❏ Andro-Teston |
| ❏ Amphedroxyn | ❏ AN-DTPA Kit |
| ❏ amphetamine | ❏ Anectine |
| ❏ Amphojel | ❏ AneuVysion Assay |
| ❏ Amphotec | ❏ Anestacon |
| ❏ amphotericin | ❏ Anesthesin |
| ❏ Ampicin | ❏ Anexsia |
| ❏ ampicillin | ❏ Angeliq |
| ❏ Ampligen | ❏ Angio Conray |
| ❏ amprenavir | ❏ Angiomax |
| ❏ amrinone lactate | ❏ Angiovist |
| ❏ Amrix | ❏ Anhydron |
| ❏ Amsustain | ❏ anidulafungin |
| ❏ Amvaz | ❏ Animi-3 |
| ❏ Amylase | ❏ Anisindione |
| ❏ amyl nitrate | ❏ anistreplase |
| ❏ Amytal Sodium | ❏ Anolor |
| ❏ Anabar | ❏ Ansaid |
| ❏ Anacel | ❏ Ansamycin |
| ❏ Anacin | ❏ Antabuse |
| ❏ Anadrol | ❏ antacids |
| ❏ Anafranil | ❏ Antagon |
| ❏ anagrelide | ❏ Antara |
| ❏ Anakinra | ❏ Antegren |
| ❏ Ana-Kit | ❏ anthelmintics |
| ❏ Analpram | ❏ anthracycline |
| ❏ ananas comosus | ❏ anthralin |
| ❏ Anaplex | ❏ AntiBetic |
| ❏ Anaprox | ❏ Antibiopto |
| ❏ Anaspaz | ❏ antihemophilic factor |
| ❏ anastrozole | ❏ antihistamines |
| ❏ Anatrast | ❏ Anti-Ige |
| ❏ Anatuss | ❏ Anti-Inhibitor |
| ❏ Anbesol | ❏ Antilirium |
| ❏ Ancef | ❏ antipyrine |
| ❏ Ancobon | ❏ antithrombin III |
| ❏ Ancrod | ❏ anti-thymocyte globulin |
| ❏ Androderm | ❏ ANTIOX |
| ❏ AndroGel | ❏ antipyrine |

| A |
|---|

- ❑ Antivenin
- ❑ Antivert
- ❑ Antizol
- ❑ Antrocol
- ❑ Anturane
- ❑ Anusol
- ❑ Anzemet
- ❑ Ao-Zidovudine
- ❑ APAP Elixer
- ❑ Apatate
- ❑ APC
- ❑ Apcitide
- ❑ Aphrodyne
- ❑ Aphthasol
- ❑ A.P.I.
- ❑ Apidra
- ❑ APL
- ❑ Aplenzin
- ❑ Apligraf
- ❑ Aplisol
- ❑ ApoA-1
- ❑ ApoA-1 Milano
- ❑ Apokyn
- ❑ apomorphine hydrochloride
- ❑ Appearex
- ❑ apraclonidine
- ❑ aprepitant
- ❑ Apriso
- ❑ Apresazide
- ❑ Apresoline
- ❑ Aprepitant
- ❑ Apri
- ❑ aprobarbital
- ❑ aprotinin
- ❑ APSAC
- ❑ Aptivus
- ❑ Aqua-Ban
- ❑ Aquachloral
- ❑ AquaLase
- ❑ AquaMEPHYTON
- ❑ Aquanil

| A |
|---|

- ❑ Aquaphor
- ❑ Aquaphyllin
- ❑ Aquasol
- ❑ Aquatar
- ❑ Aquatensen
- ❑ Aquavan
- ❑ Ara-C
- ❑ Aralast NP
- ❑ Aralen
- ❑ Aramine
- ❑ Aranesp
- ❑ Arava
- ❑ Arbutamine
- ❑ Arcalyst
- ❑ Arco-Lase
- ❑ Ardeparin
- ❑ Arduan
- ❑ Aredia
- ❑ Arestin
- ❑ Arfonad
- ❑ arformoterol tartrate
- ❑ argatroban
- ❑ ArginMax
- ❑ Aricept
- ❑ Arimidex
- ❑ aripiprazole
- ❑ Aristocort
- ❑ AristoDerm
- ❑ Aristospan
- ❑ Arixtra
- ❑ Arm-A-Med
- ❑ armodafinil
- ❑ Aromasin
- ❑ Arranon
- ❑ arsenic trioxide
- ❑ Artane
- ❑ Artecoll
- ❑ Artefill
- ❑ Arth DR
- ❑ ArthriCare
- ❑ ArthriFlex

| A | A |
|---|---|

- ❑ Arthriten
- ❑ Arthritis-Patch
- ❑ Arthro-7
- ❑ Arthrotec
- ❑ Arth-Rx
- ❑ Arthur It is
- ❑ Artiss
- ❑ Aryplase
- ❑ Asacol
- ❑ Asbron
- ❑ Ascensia Breeze
- ❑ ascorbic acid
- ❑ Ascriptin
- ❑ Asendin
- ❑ Asimia
- ❑ Asmalix
- ❑ Asmanex Twisthaler
- ❑ asparaginase
- ❑ Aspercreme
- ❑ Aspergum
- ❑ aspirin
- ❑ Astelin
- ❑ astemizole
- ❑ Astepro
- ❑ Asthmahaler
- ❑ Astragalus
- ❑ Astramorph
- ❑ Astring-O-Sol
- ❑ Atabrine
- ❑ Atacand
- ❑ Atamet
- ❑ Atapryl
- ❑ Atarax
- ❑ atazanavir
- ❑ atenolol
- ❑ Atgam
- ❑ Ativan
- ❑ ATnativ
- ❑ ATNAA
- ❑ atomoxetine HCl
- ❑ Atopiclair

- ❑ atorvastatin
- ❑ atovaquone
- ❑ ATP
- ❑ atracurium
- ❑ Atrac-Tain
- ❑ Atralin
- ❑ Atretol
- ❑ Atridox
- ❑ Atripla
- ❑ Atrohist
- ❑ Atromid-S
- ❑ AtroPen
- ❑ Atropine
- ❑ Atrosept
- ❑ Atrovent
- ❑ A/T/S
- ❑ Attapulgite
- ❑ Attenuvax
- ❑ Augmentin
- ❑ Augmentin XR
- ❑ AUK-3
- ❑ Auralgan
- ❑ auranofin
- ❑ Aureomycin
- ❑ aurothioglucose
- ❑ Auroto Otic
- ❑ Auszyme
- ❑ Authia
- ❑ Autoplex
- ❑ Avagard
- ❑ Avage
- ❑ Avalide
- ❑ Avandamet
- ❑ Avandaryl
- ❑ Avandia
- ❑ Avapro
- ❑ Avastin
- ❑ AVC
- ❑ Aveeno
- ❑ Aveenobar
- ❑ Avelox

## A

- ❑ Aventyl
- ❑ Aviane
- ❑ Avimil
- ❑ Avinza
- ❑ Avirax
- ❑ Avita
- ❑ Avlimil
- ❑ Avlosulfon
- ❑ Avobenzone
- ❑ Avodart
- ❑ Avonex
- ❑ AVX101
- ❑ Axert
- ❑ Axid
- ❑ Axocet
- ❑ Axokine
- ❑ Axotal
- ❑ Aygestin
- ❑ Ayr saline mist
- ❑ azacitidine
- ❑ Azactam
- ❑ azafluoroquinolone
- ❑ Azasan
- ❑ AzaSite
- ❑ azatadine
- ❑ Azathioprine
- ❑ Azdone
- ❑ azelaic acid
- ❑ azelastine
- ❑ Azelex
- ❑ azidothymidine
- ❑ Azilect
- ❑ azithromycin
- ❑ Azmacort
- ❑ Azo
- ❑ Azo Gantanol
- ❑ Azo Gantrisin
- ❑ Azo-Standard
- ❑ Azopt
- ❑ Azor
- ❑ AZT

## A

- ❑ aztreonam
- ❑ Azulfidine

## B

- ❑ Babylax, Fleet
- ❑ bacampicillin
- ❑ Baciquent
- ❑ Bacitracin
- ❑ Backaid
- ❑ Bacotracom
- ❑ Baclofen
- ❑ Bactine
- ❑ Bactome
- ❑ Bactocill
- ❑ Bactrim
- ❑ Bactroban
- ❑ Balagan
- ❑ Balamine
- ❑ Baldex
- ❑ Bal in oil
- ❑ balsalazide
- ❑ balsam Peru
- ❑ Baltussin
- ❑ Banan
- ❑ Bancap HC
- ❑ Band-Aid Scar
- ❑ Banflex
- ❑ Banthine
- ❑ Banzel
- ❑ Baraclude
- ❑ barbital
- ❑ barbiturates
- ❑ Baricon
- ❑ Baridol
- ❑ barium sulfate
- ❑ Barobag
- ❑ Baro-CAT
- ❑ Baroflave
- ❑ Barosperse
- ❑ Bar-test

## B

- ❑ Barotrast
- ❑ Basaljel
- ❑ basiliximab
- ❑ Baycol
- ❑ Bayer aspirin
- ❑ BayGam
- ❑ BayHep
- ❑ BayRab
- ❑ BayRho
- ❑ BayTet
- ❑ BCG vaccine
- ❑ BCNU
- ❑ BiCNU
- ❑ Beano
- ❑ Bebulin
- ❑ becaplermin
- ❑ beclomethasone
- ❑ Beclovent
- ❑ Beconase
- ❑ Beelith
- ❑ Beepen
- ❑ belladonna alkaloids
- ❑ Bellatal
- ❑ Bellergal
- ❑ benactyzine
- ❑ Benadryl
- ❑ Benadryl-D
- ❑ benazepril
- ❑ bendamustine
- ❑ bendroflumethiazide
- ❑ BeneFix
- ❑ BeneJoint
- ❑ Benemid
- ❑ Bengay
- ❑ Benicar
- ❑ Benoquin
- ❑ Benoxinate
- ❑ Bensulfoid
- ❑ bentoquatam
- ❑ Bentyl
- ❑ Benylin

## B

- ❑ Benzac
- ❑ BenzaClin gel
- ❑ Benzagel
- ❑ benzalkonium
- ❑ Benzamycin
- ❑ Benzashave
- ❑ Benzedrex
- ❑ Benzedrine
- ❑ benzethonium
- ❑ Benziq
- ❑ benzocaine
- ❑ Benzodent
- ❑ benzodiazepine
- ❑ benzoic acid
- ❑ benzonatate
- ❑ benzoyl peroxide
- ❑ benzphetamine
- ❑ benzquinamide
- ❑ benzthiazide
- ❑ benztropine mesylate
- ❑ benzydamine
- ❑ Bepadin
- ❑ bepridil
- ❑ beractant
- ❑ BeStent
- ❑ BeSure
- ❑ beta-adrenergic blockers
- ❑ beta carotene
- ❑ beta lactamase
- ❑ Betadine
- ❑ Betagan
- ❑ Betaine
- ❑ beta-lactam
- ❑ Betaloc
- ❑ betamethasone
- ❑ betamethasone dipropionate
- ❑ betamethasone valerate
- ❑ Betapace
- ❑ Betasept
- ❑ Betaseron
- ❑ Betatrex

| B |
|---|

- ❑ betaxolol
- ❑ Betaxon
- ❑ bethanechol
- ❑ Betimol
- ❑ Betoptic
- ❑ bevacizumab
- ❑ Bevitamel
- ❑ bexarotene
- ❑ Bextra
- ❑ Bexxar
- ❑ Biavax
- ❑ Biaxin
- ❑ bicalutamide
- ❑ bicarbonate of soda
- ❑ bichloracetic acid
- ❑ Bicillin
- ❑ Bicitra
- ❑ BiCNu
- ❑ BiCozene Cream
- ❑ BiDil
- ❑ bifidobacteria
- ❑ Bijuva
- ❑ Bilagog
- ❑ Bilopaque
- ❑ Biltricide
- ❑ bimatoprost
- ❑ Biocef
- ❑ Bioclate
- ❑ Bio-E-Gel
- ❑ Bio Ginkgo
- ❑ BioGlue
- ❑ Biohist
- ❑ BioLean
- ❑ BioLon
- ❑ BioMD Nutraceuticals
- ❑ Bion Tears
- ❑ Biore
- ❑ Boiron
- ❑ Bio St. John's wort
- ❑ Biotin
- ❑ Bio-Tab

| B |
|---|

- ❑ Biotest Hot-Rox
- ❑ BioThrax
- ❑ Biotin
- ❑ BioZ monitor
- ❑ Biozole
- ❑ biperiden
- ❑ biphetamine
- ❑ bisacodyl
- ❑ biskalcitrate
- ❑ bismuth subsalicylate
- ❑ bisoprolol
- ❑ bitolterol mesylate
- ❑ bivalirudin
- ❑ Black Cohash
- ❑ Blenoxane
- ❑ bleomycin
- ❑ Bleph-10
- ❑ Blephamide
- ❑ Blocadren
- ❑ B-Long
- ❑ Bluboro
- ❑ Blu-Emu
- ❑ B & O Supprettes
- ❑ Bonamil
- ❑ Bonine
- ❑ Boniva
- ❑ Bontril PDM
- ❑ Boostrix
- ❑ Borofax
- ❑ Boroleum
- ❑ bortezomib
- ❑ bosentan
- ❑ Botox
- ❑ botulinum toxin type
- ❑ BranchAmin
- ❑ Bravelle
- ❑ Breonesin
- ❑ BreathTek UBT
- ❑ Breeze2
- ❑ Brethaire
- ❑ Brethine

## B

- ❑ Bretylate
- ❑ bretylium tosylate
- ❑ Brevibloc
- ❑ Brevicon
- ❑ Brevital, sodium
- ❑ Brevoxyl
- ❑ Brexin
- ❑ briazolamide
- ❑ Bricanyl
- ❑ brimonidine
- ❑ brinzolamide
- ❑ Brioschi Powder
- ❑ Bromarest DX
- ❑ bromelain
- ❑ Bromfed
- ❑ Bromfenac
- ❑ bromocriptine
- ❑ bromonidine
- ❑ Bromo Quinine
- ❑ brompheniramine
- ❑ Bromural
- ❑ bronchodilators, adrenergic
- ❑ bronchodilators, xanthine
- ❑ Broncholate
- ❑ Bronkaid
- ❑ Bronkodyl
- ❑ Bronkometer aerosol
- ❑ Bronkosol
- ❑ Brontex
- ❑ Brovana
- ❑ brucine poison
- ❑ Bryostatin
- ❑ BSS
- ❑ buclizine
- ❑ budesonide
- ❑ bufexamac
- ❑ BufferGel
- ❑ Bufferin
- ❑ Bufopto
- ❑ Bumetanide
- ❑ Bumex

## B

- ❑ Buminate
- ❑ Bupap
- ❑ bupivacaine
- ❑ Buprenex
- ❑ buprenorphine
- ❑ bupropion
- ❑ Burn-A-Lay
- ❑ Burnicin
- ❑ Burn-Quel
- ❑ Buro-Sol
- ❑ Burow's solution
- ❑ Buserelin
- ❑ BuSpar
- ❑ buspirone
- ❑ busulfan
- ❑ busulfex
- ❑ butabarbital
- ❑ butalbital
- ❑ butaperazine
- ❑ Butazolidin
- ❑ butenafine
- ❑ Butesin
- ❑ buthiazide
- ❑ Butisol
- ❑ butoconazole
- ❑ butorphanol
- ❑ butriptyline
- ❑ butyl aminobenzoate
- ❑ butylparaben
- ❑ butynamine
- ❑ butyrophenone
- ❑ Byetta
- ❑ Bystolic

## C

- ❑ C1 Inhibitor
- ❑ caa pi
- ❑ cabergoline
- ❑ cactinomycin
- ❑ Caduet

## C

- ❑ Cafcit
- ❑ Cafergot
- ❑ caffeine
- ❑ Caladryl
- ❑ CalaGel
- ❑ Calamatum
- ❑ Calamine
- ❑ Calan
- ❑ Calcet
- ❑ Calcibind
- ❑ Calci-Chew
- ❑ calcifediol
- ❑ Calciferol
- ❑ Calcijex
- ❑ Calcimar
- ❑ Calci-Mix
- ❑ calcipotriene
- ❑ calcitonin
- ❑ Calcitonin-Salmon
- ❑ Calcitrol
- ❑ calcium
- ❑ calcium acetate
- ❑ calcium carbonate
- ❑ calcium channel blockers
- ❑ calcium chloride
- ❑ calcium citrate
- ❑ calcium disodium
- ❑ calcium gluceptate
- ❑ calcium gluconate
- ❑ Calderol
- ❑ Caldesene
- ❑ Calel-D
- ❑ calfactant
- ❑ Calm Colon
- ❑ CaloMist
- ❑ Calphosan
- ❑ Caltrate
- ❑ calvacin
- ❑ Cama Arthritis
- ❑ Camalox
- ❑ camellia sinensis

## C

- ❑ Camila
- ❑ Campath
- ❑ Campho-Phenique
- ❑ camphotamide
- ❑ Campral
- ❑ Camptosar
- ❑ camylofine
- ❑ Canasa
- ❑ Cancidas
- ❑ candesartan cilexetil
- ❑ Canesten
- ❑ Cankaid
- ❑ cannabidiol
- ❑ cannabinoid
- ❑ cannabinol
- ❑ cannabis sativa
- ❑ Cantil
- ❑ Capastat
- ❑ capecitabine
- ❑ Capex
- ❑ Capoten
- ❑ Capozide
- ❑ capreomycin
- ❑ capryloyl glycine
- ❑ capsaicin
- ❑ Captopen
- ❑ Captopril
- ❑ Captozide
- ❑ Capzasin-P
- ❑ capsicum oleoresin
- ❑ Carac cream
- ❑ Carafate
- ❑ caspofungin
- ❑ Captique
- ❑ captodiame
- ❑ captopril
- ❑ Carafate
- ❑ Carbacel
- ❑ carbachol
- ❑ carbamazepine
- ❑ carbamide peroxide

## C

- ☐ Carbamine
- ☐ Carbatrol
- ☐ carbazochrome
- ☐ Carb Cutter
- ☐ carbenicillin
- ☐ carbetapentane
- ☐ Carbex
- ☐ carbidopa/levodopa
- ☐ carbimazole
- ☐ carbinoxamine
- ☐ carbol-fuchsin paint
- ☐ carbolic acid
- ☐ carbonic anhydrase inhibitor
- ☐ carboplatin
- ☐ Carboprost
- ☐ Carboptic
- ☐ Cardene
- ☐ Cardilate
- ☐ Cardio Essentials
- ☐ CardioGen 82
- ☐ cardioplegic solution
- ☐ Cardioquin
- ☐ CardioTec Kit
- ☐ Cardiotropin
- ☐ Cardizem
- ☐ Cardura
- ☐ carisoprodol
- ☐ Carlesta
- ☐ Carmex
- ☐ carmustine
- ☐ Carnitor
- ☐ carotenoid
- ☐ carphenazine
- ☐ Cartelol
- ☐ Cartia XT
- ☐ Carrticel
- ☐ Cartrol
- ☐ carvedilol
- ☐ casanthranol
- ☐ cascara sagrada
- ☐ Casodex

## C

- ☐ caspofungin acetate
- ☐ castor oil
- ☐ Castoria
- ☐ Cataflam
- ☐ Catapres
- ☐ Catapres-TTS
- ☐ Catarase
- ☐ Catasod-Ocuxtra
- ☐ Cathflo Activase
- ☐ Catrix
- ☐ Caverject
- ☐ CAE-SCAN
- ☐ Ceclor
- ☐ Cedax
- ☐ CeeNU
- ☐ cefaclor
- ☐ cefadroxil monohydrate
- ☐ cefamandole naftate
- ☐ cefazolin
- ☐ cefdinir
- ☐ cefditoren pivoxil
- ☐ cefepime
- ☐ Cefixime
- ☐ Cefizox
- ☐ cefmetazole
- ☐ Cefobid
- ☐ Cefol Filmtab
- ☐ cefonicid
- ☐ cefoperazone
- ☐ Cefotan
- ☐ cefotaxime
- ☐ Cefotetan
- ☐ cefoxitin
- ☐ cefpodoxime
- ☐ cefprozil
- ☐ ceftazidime
- ☐ ceftibuten
- ☐ Ceftin
- ☐ ceftizoxime
- ☐ ceftriaxone
- ☐ cefuroxime

## C

- ❑ cefuroxime axetil
- ❑ Cefzil
- ❑ Celebrex
- ❑ celecoxib
- ❑ Celestone Soluspan
- ❑ Celexa
- ❑ Cellasene
- ❑ CellCept
- ❑ Cellulase
- ❑ Cellulean
- ❑ cellulose sodium phosphate
- ❑ Celluvisc lubricant
- ❑ Celontin
- ❑ Cel-U-Jec
- ❑ CenDex
- ❑ Cenestin
- ❑ Ceo-Two
- ❑ Cepacol
- ❑ cephalexin
- ❑ cephalosporins
- ❑ cephradine
- ❑ Ceprotin
- ❑ Ceptaz
- ❑ Cera
- ❑ Cerebyx
- ❑ Cerebrex
- ❑ Ceredase
- ❑ Ceredase
- ❑ Cerezyme
- ❑ cerivastatin
- ❑ Cernevit
- ❑ Cerose-DM
- ❑ Certiva
- ❑ certolizumab pegol
- ❑ Cerubidine
- ❑ Cerumenex
- ❑ Cervidil
- ❑ Cetacaine
- ❑ Cetamide
- ❑ Cetaphil
- ❑ cetirizine

## C

- ❑ Cetrorelix
- ❑ Cetrotide
- ❑ cetuximab
- ❑ cetyl alcohol
- ❑ cevimeline
- ❑ Chantix
- ❑ ChapStick
- ❑ charcoal
- ❑ Chemet
- ❑ Chenodiol
- ❑ Cheracol
- ❑ Chibroxin
- ❑ ChiRhoStim
- ❑ Chirocaine
- ❑ Chitosan
- ❑ Chlor-3
- ❑ Chloracol
- ❑ chloral hydrate
- ❑ chlorambucil
- ❑ chloramphenicol
- ❑ ChloraPrep
- ❑ Chloraseptic
- ❑ chlorcyclizine
- ❑ chlordiazepoxide
- ❑ Chloresium
- ❑ Chlorhexidine
- ❑ chlormezanone
- ❑ chloroethane
- ❑ Chlorofair
- ❑ chloroform
- ❑ Chloromycetin
- ❑ chlorophyllin
- ❑ chloroprocaine
- ❑ Chloroptic
- ❑ chloroquine
- ❑ chlorothiazide
- ❑ chloroxylenol
- ❑ chlorpheniramine
- ❑ chlorpheniramine polistirex
- ❑ chlorpromazine
- ❑ chlorpropamide

## C

- ❑ chlorprothixene
- ❑ chlorthalidone
- ❑ Chlor Trimeton
- ❑ chlorzoxazone
- ❑ Chocks vitamins
- ❑ Cholebrine
- ❑ cholecalciferol
- ❑ Choledyl
- ❑ ChoLessen
- ❑ Cholestaid
- ❑ Cholesteryl
- ❑ Cholestin
- ❑ cholestyramine
- ❑ choline bitartrate
- ❑ choline magnesium
- ❑ Cholografin
- ❑ Choloroptic
- ❑ Cholybar
- ❑ chondroitin sulfate
- ❑ Chooz
- ❑ choriogonadotropin
- ❑ chorionic gonadotropin
- ❑ Chromagen Forte
- ❑ Chroma Slim
- ❑ chromic chloride
- ❑ chromium picolinate
- ❑ chymotrypsin
- ❑ Cialis
- ❑ Cica-Care
- ❑ ciclesonide
- ❑ ciclopirox
- ❑ cidofovir
- ❑ Cilastin
- ❑ cilostazol
- ❑ Ciloxan
- ❑ cimetidine
- ❑ Cimzia
- ❑ cinacalcet
- ❑ Cinobac
- ❑ Cinoxacin
- ❑ Cipro

## C

- ❑ Cipro XR
- ❑ Ciprodex
- ❑ ciprofloxacin
- ❑ cisapride
- ❑ cisatracurium besylate
- ❑ cisplatin
- ❑ Cis-Pyro Kit
- ❑ citalopram hydrobromide
- ❑ Citracal
- ❑ CitraNatal
- ❑ citric acid
- ❑ citrocarbonate
- ❑ Citrolith
- ❑ Citrucel
- ❑ cladribine
- ❑ Claforan
- ❑ Claravis
- ❑ Clarinex
- ❑ Clarinex-D
- ❑ Claripel
- ❑ clarithromycin
- ❑ Claritin
- ❑ clavulanate
- ❑ Clean & Clear
- ❑ Clearasil
- ❑ Clear Away
- ❑ clemastine fumarate
- ❑ Clenia
- ❑ Cleocin
- ❑ clevidipine
- ❑ Cleviprex
- ❑ Clidinium
- ❑ Climara
- ❑ Climara Pro
- ❑ Clinac
- ❑ Clinda-Derm
- ❑ Clindagel
- ❑ clindamycin
- ❑ clindamycin hydrochloride
- ❑ clindamycin phosphate
- ❑ Clindesse

## C

- Clindets Pledgets
- Clindex
- Clinimix
- Clinoril
- Clinoxide
- Clioquinol
- clobetasol
- clobetasol propionate
- Clobevate
- Clobex
- clocortolone pivalate
- clofarabine
- Clolar
- Clorpactin WES 90
- Clocream
- Cloderm
- Clofazimine
- clofibrate
- Clomid
- clomiphene
- clomipramine
- clonazepam
- clonidine
- clonidine hydrochloride
- clopidogrel
- clorazepate
- Clorpactin WCS
- Clorpres
- clotrimazole
- cloxacillin
- Cloxapen
- clozapine
- Clozaril
- CM Plex
- CMV-IGIV
- cod liver oil
- Codamine
- codeine
- Codeprex
- Codiclear DH
- Codimal DM

## C

- Codrix
- Coenzyme Q-10
- Cogentin
- Cognex
- Colazal
- Colace
- Colazal
- ColBENEMID
- colchicine
- Coldcalm
- Cold-EEZE
- colesevelam
- Colestid
- colestipol
- colfosceril
- colistimethate
- colistin sulfate
- Collagenase
- Collyrium
- Colocort
- Coly-Mycin
- Colyte
- Comax
- Combigan
- CombiPatch
- Combipres
- Combivent
- Combivir
- Combunox
- Commit
- Compazine
- Compound W
- Compro
- Comtan
- Comtrex
- Comvax
- Conceptrol
- Concerta
- Condylox
- Congess
- Congespirin

## C

- ☐ conivaptan
- ☐ conjugated estrogen
- ☐ Conray
- ☐ Constant-T
- ☐ Contac
- ☐ Contac-D
- ☐ Copaxone
- ☐ Copegus
- ☐ copper
- ☐ CoQ10
- ☐ Coquinone
- ☐ Coramine
- ☐ Cordarone
- ☐ Cordran
- ☐ Cordran tape
- ☐ cordyceps sinensis
- ☐ Cordymax CS
- ☐ Coreg
- ☐ Corgard
- ☐ Coricidin
- ☐ Coricidin HBP
- ☐ corium
- ☐ Corlopam
- ☐ cormax
- ☐ Corophyllin
- ☐ Correctol
- ☐ Cortaid
- ☐ Cortane-B Otic
- ☐ Cortef
- ☐ Cortenema
- ☐ Cortic ear drops
- ☐ corticorelin
- ☐ corticotropin
- ☐ Cortifoam
- ☐ cortisol
- ☐ cortisone
- ☐ Cortisporin
- ☐ Cortitrol
- ☐ Cortizone-10
- ☐ Cortone
- ☐ Cortrosyn

## C

- ☐ Corvert
- ☐ Corzide
- ☐ Cosamin
- ☐ Cosmegen
- ☐ CosmoDerm
- ☐ CosmoPlast
- ☐ Cosopt
- ☐ cosyntropin
- ☐ Cotanal
- ☐ Cotara
- ☐ Cotazym
- ☐ Co-trimoxazole
- ☐ CoTylenol
- ☐ Coumadin
- ☐ Covera-HS
- ☐ COX-2 inhibitor
- ☐ Cozaar
- ☐ creatine phosphate
- ☐ Creomulsion
- ☐ Creon
- ☐ Crestor
- ☐ Crinone
- ☐ Crixivan
- ☐ Crolom
- ☐ cromolyn sodium
- ☐ Cromoptic
- ☐ crotamiton
- ☐ Cruex
- ☐ Cryselle
- ☐ Crystodigin
- ☐ Cubicin
- ☐ cupric chloride
- ☐ Cuprimine
- ☐ Curad Scar Therapy
- ☐ Cura-Heat
- ☐ Curosurf
- ☐ Custodiol HTK
- ☐ Cutivate
- ☐ CX-516
- ☐ cyanocobalamin
- ☐ Cyanokit

## C

- ❑ Cyclen
- ❑ Cyclessa
- ❑ cyclobarbital
- ❑ cyclobenzaprine
- ❑ Cyclocort
- ❑ Cycloflex
- ❑ Cyclogyl
- ❑ Cyclokapron
- ❑ Cyclomydril
- ❑ cyclopentobarbital
- ❑ cyclopentolate
- ❑ cyclophosphamide
- ❑ cycloserine
- ❑ cyclosporine
- ❑ cyclothiazide
- ❑ Cycrin
- ❑ Cylert
- ❑ Cymbalta
- ❑ Cynara-SL
- ❑ Cinryze
- ❑ Cypher stent
- ❑ cyproheptadine
- ❑ cyproterone
- ❑ Cystadane
- ❑ Cystagon
- ❑ cysteamine
- ❑ Cysto-Conray
- ❑ Cystographin
- ❑ Cystospaz
- ❑ Cytadren
- ❑ cytarabine
- ❑ CytoGam
- ❑ cytomegalovirus vaccine
- ❑ Cytomel
- ❑ Cyto Prep
- ❑ Cytosar-U
- ❑ Cytotec
- ❑ Cytovene
- ❑ Cytoxan

## D

- ❑ D.A. Chewable
- ❑ D.A. Tablets
- ❑ DHA
- ❑ DHEA
- ❑ DDAVP
- ❑ D.H.E. 45
- ❑ DML
- ❑ Dtic-Dome
- ❑ Dacarbazine
- ❑ Daclizumab
- ❑ Dacogen
- ❑ Dacriose
- ❑ dactinomycin
- ❑ Dalalone
- ❑ dalfopristin
- ❑ Dalgin
- ❑ Dallergy
- ❑ Dalmane
- ❑ dalteparin sodium
- ❑ Damason-P
- ❑ danazol
- ❑ danaparoid
- ❑ Danocrine
- ❑ Dantrium
- ❑ dantrolene
- ❑ dapiprazole
- ❑ dapsone
- ❑ Daptacel
- ❑ daptomycin
- ❑ Daranide
- ❑ Daraprim
- ❑ darbepoetin alfa
- ❑ darifenacin
- ❑ Dartal
- ❑ darunavir
- ❑ Darvocet-A 500
- ❑ Darvocet-N
- ❑ Darvon
- ❑ dasatinib
- ❑ Datril

## D

- ❑ daunorubicin
- ❑ Daunoxome
- ❑ DawnMist
- ❑ Daypro
- ❑ DayQuil
- ❑ Daytrana
- ❑ DCF
- ❑ DDAVP
- ❑ ddC
- ❑ Debrox
- ❑ Decadron
- ❑ Deca-Durabolin
- ❑ Decaject
- ❑ Decaspray
- ❑ decitabine
- ❑ Declomycin
- ❑ Deconamine
- ❑ Deconsal
- ❑ Decubitene
- ❑ Defen-LA
- ❑ deferasirox
- ❑ deferoxamine mesylate
- ❑ Definity
- ❑ Degarelix
- ❑ Degest
- ❑ dehydro-epiandrosterone
- ❑ Delatest injection
- ❑ Delatestryl
- ❑ delavirdine
- ❑ Delcid
- ❑ Delestrogen
- ❑ Delfen
- ❑ Delsym
- ❑ Deltasone
- ❑ Demadex
- ❑ demecarium bromide
- ❑ demeclocycline
- ❑ Demerol
- ❑ Demi-Groton
- ❑ Demser
- ❑ Demulen

## D

- ❑ Denavir
- ❑ denileukin diftitox
- ❑ Denorex
- ❑ Dentapaine
- ❑ DentiPatch
- ❑ Dent-Zel-Ite
- ❑ Depacon
- ❑ Depade
- ❑ Depakene
- ❑ Depakote
- ❑ depAndro injection
- ❑ Depen
- ❑ DepoCyt
- ❑ DepoDur
- ❑ DepoFoam
- ❑ Depo-Medrol
- ❑ Depomorphine
- ❑ Deponit
- ❑ Depo Provera
- ❑ Depotest injection
- ❑ depo-subQ provera
- ❑ Depo-Testosterone
- ❑ deprenyl
- ❑ Derifil
- ❑ Dermacil tape
- ❑ Dermarest
- ❑ Derma-Smoothe
- ❑ Dermatop
- ❑ DermOtic Oil
- ❑ Desenex
- ❑ Desferal
- ❑ desflurane
- ❑ desipramine
- ❑ Desirudin
- ❑ Desitin
- ❑ desloratadine
- ❑ desmopressin
- ❑ Desogen
- ❑ desogestrel
- ❑ Desonate
- ❑ desonide

## D

- ❑ DesOwen
- ❑ desoximetasone
- ❑ Desoxyn
- ❑ Despec
- ❑ Desquam-E
- ❑ desvenlafaxine
- ❑ Desyrel
- ❑ detemir
- ❑ Detrol
- ❑ Detrol LA
- ❑ Devonex
- ❑ Dexacort
- ❑ dexamethasone
- ❑ Dexatrim
- ❑ dexbrompheniramine
- ❑ dexchlorpheniramine
- ❑ dexmedetomidine
- ❑ dexmethylphenidate
- ❑ Dexedrine
- ❑ DexFerrum
- ❑ Dexone
- ❑ Dexpak
- ❑ dexrazoxane
- ❑ dextran-70
- ❑ dextroamphetamine sulfate
- ❑ dextromethorphan
- ❑ dextrose
- ❑ Dextrostat
- ❑ Dezocine
- ❑ DHA
- ❑ DHE-45
- ❑ DHS tar shampoo
- ❑ DHT Intensol
- ❑ DiaBeta
- ❑ Diabet-X
- ❑ Diabe-Tuss DM
- ❑ Diabinese
- ❑ Dialose
- ❑ Diamox
- ❑ Diamox Sequels
- ❑ Dianeal

## D

- ❑ Diastat
- ❑ diatrizoate
- ❑ diatrizoic acid
- ❑ diazepam
- ❑ diazoxide
- ❑ Dibenzyline
- ❑ DiBromm
- ❑ Dicarbosil
- ❑ dichloralphenazone
- ❑ dichlorphenamide
- ❑ diclofenac epolamine
- ❑ diclofenac potassium
- ❑ diclofenac sodium
- ❑ Dicloxacillin
- ❑ dicyclomine
- ❑ didanosine
- ❑ Didrex
- ❑ Didronel
- ❑ dienestrol
- ❑ diethylpropion
- ❑ diethylstilbestrol diphosphate
- ❑ difenoxin
- ❑ Differin
- ❑ Diff-Quick Stain
- ❑ diflorasone
- ❑ Diflucan
- ❑ Diflunisal
- ❑ difluprednate
- ❑ Di-Gel
- ❑ Digibind
- ❑ Digitek
- ❑ digoxin
- ❑ digoxin immune fab
- ❑ dihydrocodeine
- ❑ dihydroergotamine
- ❑ dihydrotachysterol
- ❑ diiodohydroxyquin
- ❑ Dilacor
- ❑ Dilantin
- ❑ Dilatrate-SR
- ❑ Dilaudid

| D | D |
|---|---|

- [ ] Dilor
- [ ] Dilitia
- [ ] Diltiazem
- [ ] Diluent
- [ ] dimenhydrinate
- [ ] Dimetane-DX
- [ ] Dimetapp
- [ ] dimethicone
- [ ] dimethyl sulfoxide
- [ ] Dinate
- [ ] dinoprostone
- [ ] dioctyl sodium
- [ ] DioMedicone
- [ ] Diovan
- [ ] dioxybenzone
- [ ] Dipentum
- [ ] diphenhydramine
- [ ] diphenidol
- [ ] diphenoxylate
- [ ] diphenylhydantoin
- [ ] diphtheria CRM
- [ ] Dipivefrin
- [ ] dipotassium phosphate
- [ ] Diprivan
- [ ] Diprolene
- [ ] Diprosone
- [ ] dipyridamole
- [ ] diquafosol tetrasodium
- [ ] dirithromycin
- [ ] Disalcid
- [ ] Dismutax
- [ ] Disobrom
- [ ] disodium phosphate
- [ ] disopyramide phosphate
- [ ] Disotate
- [ ] DisperMox
- [ ] disulfiram
- [ ] Ditropan
- [ ] Ditropan-XL
- [ ] Diucardin
- [ ] Diuchlor

- [ ] Diulo
- [ ] Diupres
- [ ] Diurex
- [ ] Diuril
- [ ] divalproex sodium
- [ ] Divigel
- [ ] DMARDS
- [ ] DML
- [ ] DMSO
- [ ] Doan's
- [ ] Dobutamine
- [ ] Dobutrex
- [ ] docetaxel
- [ ] docosahexaenoic acid
- [ ] docusate sodium
- [ ] Docusol
- [ ] Dofetilide
- [ ] dolasetron mesylate
- [ ] Dolobid
- [ ] Dolophine
- [ ] Dolorac
- [ ] Domeboro
- [ ] Donatussin
- [ ] donepezil
- [ ] Dong Quai
- [ ] Donnagel
- [ ] Donnatal
- [ ] Donnazyme
- [ ] Dopamine
- [ ] Dopram
- [ ] Doral
- [ ] Dorbane
- [ ] Dorbantyl
- [ ] Doribax
- [ ] Doriden
- [ ] doripenem
- [ ] dornase alfa
- [ ] Doryx
- [ ] dorzolamide
- [ ] Dosaflex
- [ ] Dostinex

## D

- ❑ DoubleCap
- ❑ Doubtrex
- ❑ Dovonex
- ❑ doxacurium
- ❑ doxapram
- ❑ doxazosin
- ❑ doxepin
- ❑ doxercalciferol
- ❑ Doxidan
- ❑ Doxil
- ❑ Doxorubicin
- ❑ Doxy 100
- ❑ doxychel hyclate
- ❑ doxycycline calcium
- ❑ doxycycline hyclate
- ❑ doxycycline monohydrate
- ❑ doxylamine succinate
- ❑ Drabinol
- ❑ Dramamine
- ❑ Dramanate
- ❑ Drinalfa
- ❑ Dristan
- ❑ Drithrocreme
- ❑ Drixoral
- ❑ Dronabinol
- ❑ Droperidol
- ❑ drospirenone
- ❑ Drotrecogin Alfa
- ❑ Droxia
- ❑ drug-eluting stent
- ❑ Drysol
- ❑ Dryvax
- ❑ DTIC-DOME
- ❑ Duac
- ❑ Duet Stuartnatal
- ❑ Duetact
- ❑ Duagen
- ❑ Dulcodos
- ❑ Dulcolax
- ❑ duloxetine
- ❑ DuoFilm

## D

- ❑ Duo-Medihaler
- ❑ DuoNeb
- ❑ DuoVisc
- ❑ Duphalic
- ❑ Duracef
- ❑ Duraclon
- ❑ Duract
- ❑ Duradrin
- ❑ Duragesic
- ❑ Dura-Gest
- ❑ Duramorph
- ❑ Duranest
- ❑ Duraphyl
- ❑ Dura-Tap/PD
- ❑ Duratest
- ❑ Durathate
- ❑ Duratuss
- ❑ Dura-Vent
- ❑ Duretic
- ❑ Durezol
- ❑ Duricef
- ❑ Dutasteride
- ❑ Dyazide
- ❑ Dyclone
- ❑ dyclonine
- ❑ Dyflex
- ❑ Dylix
- ❑ Dymelor
- ❑ Dymenate
- ❑ Dynabac
- ❑ Dynacin
- ❑ Dynacirc
- ❑ Dynapen
- ❑ dyphylline
- ❑ dypridamole
- ❑ Dyrenium
- ❑ Dytuss

## E

- ❑ E2F Decoy

| E | E |
|---|---|

- ❑ EAS Thermo DynamX
- ❑ Easprin
- ❑ Easypod
- ❑ E-Carpine
- ❑ Echinacea
- ❑ Echodide
- ❑ echothiophate iodide
- ❑ EC-Naprosyn
- ❑ econazole
- ❑ Econochlor
- ❑ Econopred
- ❑ Ecostatin
- ❑ Ecotrin
- ❑ eculizumab
- ❑ Edecrin
- ❑ EdemeX
- ❑ Edetate [EDTA]
- ❑ Edex
- ❑ edrophonium
- ❑ EDTA
- ❑ E.E.S.
- ❑ Efacor
- ❑ efalizumab
- ❑ efavirenz
- ❑ Effexor XR
- ❑ eflornithine
- ❑ Efricel
- ❑ Efroxine
- ❑ Efudex
- ❑ E-Gems
- ❑ eicosapentaenoic acid
- ❑ ELA-Max
- ❑ Elaprase
- ❑ Elavil
- ❑ Eldepryl
- ❑ Eldercaps
- ❑ Eldertonic
- ❑ Eldopaque
- ❑ Eldoquin
- ❑ Elecare
- ❑ Elestat

- ❑ Elestrin
- ❑ Eletone cream
- ❑ Eletriptan
- ❑ Elevess
- ❑ Elexon
- ❑ Elidel cream
- ❑ Eligard
- ❑ Elimite
- ❑ Elitek
- ❑ Elixicon
- ❑ Elixomin
- ❑ Elixophyllin
- ❑ ElixSure
- ❑ Ellence
- ❑ Elmiron
- ❑ Elocon
- ❑ Eloxatin
- ❑ Elspar
- ❑ eltrombopag
- ❑ Emadine
- ❑ Embeline
- ❑ Embrex 600
- ❑ Emcodeine
- ❑ Emcyt
- ❑ Emdogain
- ❑ emedastine
- ❑ Emend
- ❑ Emergen-C
- ❑ Emetrol
- ❑ Emgel
- ❑ Eminase
- ❑ EMLA anesthetic disc
- ❑ Empirin
- ❑ Emsam
- ❑ emtricitabine
- ❑ Emtriva
- ❑ E-Mycin
- ❑ Enablex
- ❑ enalapril
- ❑ enalaprilat
- ❑ Enbrel

| E | E |
|---|---|
| ❏ Encainide | ❏ epinastine hydrochloride |
| ❏ Endal-HD | ❏ epinephrine |
| ❏ Endantadine | ❏ EpiPen Auto-Injector |
| ❏ Endeavor | ❏ EpiPen Jr |
| ❏ Endocet | ❏ epirubicin |
| ❏ Endodan | ❏ Epitol |
| ❏ Endometrin | ❏ Epitope OraSure |
| ❏ Endrate | ❏ Epitrate |
| ❏ Enduron | ❏ Epivir |
| ❏ Enecat | ❏ Epivir-HBV |
| ❏ Enfamil Natalins RX | ❏ eplerenone |
| ❏ enflurane | ❏ eletriptan |
| ❏ enfuvirtide | ❏ eplernone |
| ❏ Engerix-B | ❏ Epoetin Alfa |
| ❏ Enhanze SC | ❏ Epogen |
| ❏ Enjuvia | ❏ epolamine |
| ❏ Enlon | ❏ epoprostenol |
| ❏ Enoxacin | ❏ Epothilone |
| ❏ enoxaparin | ❏ Eppy |
| ❏ Enpresse | ❏ epratuzumab |
| ❏ entacapone | ❏ Eprex |
| ❏ entecavir | ❏ eprosartan mesylate |
| ❏ Entereg | ❏ eptifibatide |
| ❏ Enteryx | ❏ Epzicom |
| ❏ Entex | ❏ Equagesic |
| ❏ Entocort | ❏ Equalactin |
| ❏ Entrobar | ❏ Equanil |
| ❏ ENTSOL | ❏ Equetro |
| ❏ Enydrial | ❏ Eraxis |
| ❏ Enzyte | ❏ Erbitux |
| ❏ Eovist | ❏ Ercaf |
| ❏ EPA | ❏ Ergamisol |
| ❏ Ephedra | ❏ ergocalciferol |
| ❏ ephedrine | ❏ ergolid mesylate |
| ❏ Epi-C | ❏ Ergomar |
| ❏ Epiduo | ❏ ergonovine |
| ❏ Epifoam | ❏ ergotamine |
| ❏ Epifrin | ❏ Ergotrate Maleate |
| ❏ E-Pilo | ❏ erlotinib |
| ❏ Epimorph | ❏ Errin |
| ❏ Epinal | ❏ Ertaczo |

| E | E |
|---|---|

- ❑ ertapenem
- ❑ ERYC
- ❑ Erycette
- ❑ Erygel
- ❑ Ery-Max
- ❑ Eryped
- ❑ Ery-Tab
- ❑ Erythrocin
- ❑ erythromycin ethylsuccinate
- ❑ erythropoietin
- ❑ Eryzole
- ❑ escitalopram oxalate
- ❑ Esclim
- ❑ Eserin
- ❑ Esgic
- ❑ Esidrix
- ❑ Esimil
- ❑ Eskalith
- ❑ esmolol
- ❑ esomeprazole
- ❑ Essiac tea
- ❑ estazolam
- ❑ esterase
- ❑ Estinyl
- ❑ Estorra
- ❑ Estrace
- ❑ Estraderm
- ❑ estradiol
- ❑ estradiol acetate
- ❑ estradiol cypionate
- ❑ estradiol valerate
- ❑ estramustine phosphate
- ❑ Estratab
- ❑ Estratest
- ❑ Estratest H.S.
- ❑ Estrin-D
- ❑ Estring vaginal ring
- ❑ Estrocare
- ❑ EstroGel
- ❑ estrogen
- ❑ estrogen, conjugated

- ❑ estrogen, esterified
- ❑ estropipate
- ❑ Estrasorb
- ❑ Estrostep 21
- ❑ Estrostep FE
- ❑ eszopiclone
- ❑ etanercept
- ❑ ethacrynate sodium
- ❑ ethacrynic acid
- ❑ ethambutol
- ❑ Ethamolin
- ❑ ethanolamine oleate
- ❑ ethchlorvynol
- ❑ ether
- ❑ ethinyl estradiol
- ❑ ethiodized oil
- ❑ Ethiodol
- ❑ ethionamide
- ❑ Ethmozine
- ❑ ethosuximide
- ❑ Ethrane
- ❑ ethyl aminobenzoate
- ❑ ethyl chloride
- ❑ ethylbenztropine
- ❑ ethynodiol diacetate
- ❑ Ethyol
- ❑ etidocaine
- ❑ etidronate disodium
- ❑ etodolac
- ❑ etonogestrel
- ❑ Etopophos
- ❑ etoposide
- ❑ etozolin
- ❑ Etrafon
- ❑ etravirine
- ❑ etretinate
- ❑ ETS
- ❑ eucalyptus
- ❑ Eucerin
- ❑ Eugenol
- ❑ Euglucon

## E

- Eulexin
- Eurax
- Evac-Q-Kwik
- Evac
- Evactol
- EvaMist
- Everone
- Exforge
- Evicel
- Evista
- Evithrom
- Evoclin
- Evolence
- Evoxac
- Exanta
- Excedrin
- Excedrin Quicktabs
- Exelon
- Exemestane
- Exenatide
- exendin-4
- Exforge
- Exgest
- Exisulind
- Exjade
- Ex-Lax
- Exna
- Exosurf
- Exsel
- Extendryl
- Extina
- Extraneal
- Extrasorb
- Exubera
- EYRC
- Eyesine
- Eye Stream
- EZ-Char
- ezetimibe
- EZ Med Test
- E-Z Spacer

## F

- Fabrazyme
- Factive
- factor IX
- Factrel
- famciclovir
- famotidine
- Famvir
- Fansidar
- Fareston
- Faslodex
- Fastin
- fat emulsions
- FazaClo
- FDS feminine spray
- FEIBA VH
- Felbamate
- Felbatol
- Feldene
- felodipine
- Femara
- Fem-Cap
- FemCare
- Femcet
- Femcon FE
- Femepizole
- Femhrt
- Femizole
- Fempatch
- Femring
- Femstat
- Femtrace
- Fenesin
- fenofibrate
- fenofibric
- Fenoglide
- fenoldopam
- fenoprofen
- Fen-Phen
- fentanyl
- Fentora
- Feosol

| F | F |
|---|---|
| ❑ Fero-Folic | ❑ Flolan |
| ❑ Fero-Grad | ❑ Flomax |
| ❑ Ferralet | ❑ Flonase |
| ❑ Ferrlecit | ❑ Flo-Pred |
| ❑ ferrous fumarate | ❑ Florical |
| ❑ ferrous gluconate | ❑ Florinef |
| ❑ ferrous sulfate | ❑ Florone |
| ❑ Fertinex | ❑ Floropryl |
| ❑ fesoterodine fumarate | ❑ Florvite |
| ❑ Fe-Tinic | ❑ Flovent |
| ❑ Fetrin | ❑ Flovent Diskus |
| ❑ fexofenadine | ❑ Floxin |
| ❑ fiber | ❑ floxuridine |
| ❑ FiberCon | ❑ Fluarix |
| ❑ Fibrinase | ❑ Fluclox |
| ❑ fibrin sealant [Tisseel VH] | ❑ fluconazole |
| ❑ filgrastim | ❑ flucytosine |
| ❑ Finacea | ❑ Fludara |
| ❑ finasteride | ❑ fludarabine |
| ❑ Finevin cream | ❑ fludeoxyglucose F-18 |
| ❑ Fioricet | ❑ fludrocortisones |
| ❑ Fiorinal | ❑ FluLaval |
| ❑ Fiorpap | ❑ Flumadine |
| ❑ Fiortal | ❑ flumazenil |
| ❑ Flagyl | ❑ FluMist |
| ❑ flavocoxid | ❑ flunisolide |
| ❑ flavoxate | ❑ flunitrazepam |
| ❑ Flebogamma | ❑ fluocinolone |
| ❑ flecainide | ❑ fluocinonide |
| ❑ Flector | ❑ Fluogen |
| ❑ Fleet Anorectal | ❑ Fluonid |
| ❑ Fleet Babylax | ❑ Fluoracaine |
| ❑ Fleet Bisacodyl | ❑ fluorescein |
| ❑ Fleet Enema | ❑ Fluorescite |
| ❑ Fleet Pedia-Lax | ❑ Fluoreseptic |
| ❑ Fleet Phospho-Soda | ❑ Fluorets |
| ❑ Fletcher's Castoria | ❑ Flouri-Methane |
| ❑ Flex-a-min | ❑ fluorometholone |
| ❑ Flexbumin | ❑ Fluoroplex |
| ❑ Flexeril | ❑ fluoroquinolone |
| ❑ Flexoject | ❑ fluorouracil |

| **F** | **F** |
|---|---|
| ❑ Fluothane | ❑ Fortaz |
| ❑ fluoxetine | ❑ Forteo |
| ❑ fluoxymesterone | ❑ Fortical |
| ❑ fluphenazine | ❑ Fortigel |
| ❑ flurandrenolide | ❑ Fortovase |
| ❑ flurazepam | ❑ Fosamax |
| ❑ flurbiprofen | ❑ fosamprenavir |
| ❑ Fluress | ❑ fosaprepitant dimeglumine |
| ❑ Fluro-Ethyl | ❑ foscarnet |
| ❑ FluShield | ❑ Foscavir |
| ❑ fluspirilene | ❑ fosfomycin |
| ❑ fluticasone | ❑ Fosfree |
| ❑ fluticasone furoate | ❑ fosinopril |
| ❑ flutamide | ❑ fosphenytoin |
| ❑ fluvastatin | ❑ fospropofol |
| ❑ Fluvirin | ❑ Fosrenol |
| ❑ fluvoxamine | ❑ Fosteum |
| ❑ Fluxid | ❑ Fo-Ti |
| ❑ Fluzone | ❑ Fototar |
| ❑ FML | ❑ Fragmin |
| ❑ Focalin | ❑ Framycetin |
| ❑ Folex | ❑ FreAmine |
| ❑ Folgard | ❑ FreeLax |
| ❑ folic acid | ❑ Frova |
| ❑ folinic acid | ❑ frovatriptan succinate |
| ❑ Follistim | ❑ FUDR |
| ❑ Follistim/Antagon Kit | ❑ Ful-Glo |
| ❑ follitropin alfa | ❑ Fulvestrant |
| ❑ follitropin beta | ❑ Fulvicin |
| ❑ Folvite | ❑ Fumatinic |
| ❑ fomepizole | ❑ Funduscein |
| ❑ Fomivirsen | ❑ FungiClear |
| ❑ Fondaparinux sodium | ❑ FungiCure |
| ❑ Foradil | ❑ Fungizone |
| ❑ Forane | ❑ Fungoid creme |
| ❑ Formadon | ❑ Furacin |
| ❑ formaldehyde | ❑ Furadantin |
| ❑ Formalin | ❑ Furane |
| ❑ formoterol fumarate | ❑ furazolidone |
| ❑ formoterol fumarate dihydrate | ❑ Furosemide |
| ❑ Fortamet | ❑ Furoxone |

## F

- ❏ fusion inhibitors
- ❏ Fuzeon

## G

- ❏ gaba analog
- ❏ gabapentin
- ❏ Gabitril
- ❏ Gadodiamide
- ❏ gadofosveset
- ❏ gadolinium
- ❏ gadoteridol
- ❏ gadoversetamide
- ❏ gadoxetate
- ❏ gallamine triethiodide
- ❏ galantamine
- ❏ gallium nitrate
- ❏ galsulfase
- ❏ Galzin
- ❏ gamma hydroxybutryic acid
- ❏ Gamimune
- ❏ Gammagard
- ❏ Gammar-P
- ❏ gamma vinyl-GABA
- ❏ Gamunex
- ❏ ganciclovir
- ❏ Ganirelix
- ❏ Ganite
- ❏ ganoderma lucinum
- ❏ Gantanol
- ❏ Gantrisin
- ❏ Garamycin
- ❏ Gardasil
- ❏ GasAid
- ❏ Gastrocrom
- ❏ Gastrografin
- ❏ GastroMark
- ❏ Gastroview
- ❏ Gas-X
- ❏ gatifloxacin
- ❏ Gaviscon

## G

- ❏ GBH
- ❏ Gebauer's ethyl chloride
- ❏ Gefitinib
- ❏ Gelcid
- ❏ Gelfilm
- ❏ Gelfoam
- ❏ Gel-Ose
- ❏ Gelpirin
- ❏ Gelusil
- ❏ gemcitabine
- ❏ gemfibrozil
- ❏ gemifloxacin mesylate
- ❏ gemtuzumab
- ❏ Gemzar
- ❏ Gen-XENE
- ❏ Gen-Glybe
- ❏ Genapax
- ❏ GenCept
- ❏ GenESA
- ❏ Gengraf
- ❏ genistein aglycone
- ❏ Genoptic
- ❏ Genora
- ❏ Genotropin
- ❏ Gentak
- ❏ Gentamicin
- ❏ GenTeal
- ❏ gentian violet
- ❏ Gentlax
- ❏ GentleWave
- ❏ Gentran 40
- ❏ genzyme
- ❏ Geocillin
- ❏ Geodon
- ❏ Geopen
- ❏ Geref
- ❏ Gerimed
- ❏ Geriplex
- ❏ Geritol
- ❏ Geroton
- ❏ Gero-Vita

| **G** | **G** |
|---|---|
| ❏ Gevrabon | ❏ glycine |
| ❏ Gevral | ❏ glycopyrrolate |
| ❏ GHB | ❏ glycyrrhetinic acid |
| ❏ ginkgo biloba | ❏ Glynase |
| ❏ Ginkoba | ❏ Glynase Prestab |
| ❏ Ginkogin | ❏ Gly-Oxide |
| ❏ Ginseng | ❏ Glyquin cream |
| ❏ Glandosane | ❏ Glysenid |
| ❏ glatiramer | ❏ Glyset |
| ❏ Glaucofit | ❏ Glyvic |
| ❏ Glaucon | ❏ G-mycetin |
| ❏ Glauma | ❏ Gold Bond |
| ❏ Gleevec | ❏ gold sodium thiomalate |
| ❏ Gliadel | ❏ GoLYTELY |
| ❏ glimepiride | ❏ gonadorelin |
| ❏ glipizide | ❏ gonadotropin |
| ❏ globulin | ❏ Gonak |
| ❏ Glofil-125 | ❏ Gonal-F |
| ❏ Gluca-Balance | ❏ Gordochom |
| ❏ GlucaGen | ❏ goserelin acetate |
| ❏ Glucagon [rDNA origin] | ❏ gramicidin |
| ❏ Glucamide | ❏ granisetron |
| ❏ Glucerna | ❏ Granulex |
| ❏ glucono-delta lactone | ❏ Gravol |
| ❏ Glucophage | ❏ grepafloxacin |
| ❏ glucosamine sulfate | ❏ Grifulvin V |
| ❏ glucose oxidase | ❏ Grisactin |
| ❏ glucose polymer | ❏ griseofulvin |
| ❏ Glucotrol | ❏ Gris-Peg |
| ❏ Glucovance | ❏ Guaifed |
| ❏ glulisine | ❏ guaifenesin |
| ❏ Glumetza | ❏ Guaimax |
| ❏ Glusamin | ❏ guaifenex |
| ❏ glutamine | ❏ Guai-Vent/PSE |
| ❏ glutathione | ❏ guanabenz |
| ❏ Glutofac | ❏ Guanadrel |
| ❏ Glutose | ❏ Guanethidine |
| ❏ glyburide | ❏ guanfacine |
| ❏ glycerin | ❏ Guanidine |
| ❏ glyceryl guaiacolate | ❏ Guayanesin |
| ❏ glyceryl trinitrate | ❏ guiatuss |

## G

- ❑ GVG
- ❑ Gynazole
- ❑ Gynecare ThermaChoice
- ❑ Gyne-Lotrimin
- ❑ Gyne-Trosyd
- ❑ Gynix
- ❑ Gynodiol
- ❑ Gynol II

## H

- ❑ H5NI
- ❑ Habitrol
- ❑ haemophilius beta
- ❑ halcinonide
- ❑ Halcion
- ❑ Haldol
- ❑ Haley's M-O
- ❑ Halfan
- ❑ HalfLytely
- ❑ Halfprin
- ❑ halobetasol propionate
- ❑ halofantrine
- ❑ halog
- ❑ haloperidol
- ❑ Halotestin
- ❑ Halothane
- ❑ Halotussin AC syrup
- ❑ Havrix
- ❑ hawafena
- ❑ H-BIG
- ❑ HD 85
- ❑ HD 200 Plus
- ❑ Head & Shoulders
- ❑ Healthprin
- ❑ Hectorol
- ❑ Heet
- ❑ Helicosol
- ❑ Helidac therapy
- ❑ Helixate
- ❑ Helizide

## H

- ❑ Hemabate
- ❑ Hemaspan
- ❑ HemCon Bandage
- ❑ hemin
- ❑ Hemocyte
- ❑ Hemofil
- ❑ Hemorid
- ❑ Hemril suppositories
- ❑ Hemspray
- ❑ HepaGam B
- ❑ Hepalean
- ❑ Heparin
- ❑ Heparine
- ❑ HepatAmine
- ❑ Hep-B-Gammagee
- ❑ Hep-Forte
- ❑ Hep-Lock
- ❑ Hepsera
- ❑ heptabarb
- ❑ HER2/neu
- ❑ Herceptin
- ❑ Herpecin-L
- ❑ Herpetrol
- ❑ Herplex
- ❑ HES
- ❑ Hespan
- ❑ Hetastarch
- ❑ Hexabrix
- ❑ Hexadrol
- ❑ Hexalen
- ❑ Hibiclens
- ❑ Hibistat
- ❑ HibTITER
- ❑ Hismanal
- ❑ Histalet
- ❑ Histatrol
- ❑ Histerone
- ❑ Histinex
- ❑ histrelin
- ❑ Histussin HC
- ❑ Hivid

## H

- HMG-CoA Reductase inhibitor
- HMS
- homatropine
- homocysteine
- homosalate
- Honvol
- HPA-23
- HP Acthar
- Humalog – pen and Kwikpen
- Humate
- Humate-P
- Humatrope
- Humegon
- Humibid
- Humira
- Humorsol
- Humulin 50/50
- Humulin 70/30
- Humulin N
- Humulin R
- Hurricaine
- Hyalgan
- hyaluronate
- hyaluronic acid
- hyaluronidase
- Hyate
- Hycamtin
- HYcet
- Hycodan
- Hycomine
- Hyco-Pap
- Hycosin
- Hycotuss
- Hydeltra
- Hydeltrasol
- Hydergine
- hydralazine
- hydralazine hydrochloride
- Hydrate
- Hydra-Zide
- hydrazine

## H

- Hydrea
- Hydrex
- Hydrisalic gel
- Hydrisinol creme
- Hydrocet
- Hydrocil
- Hydrochlorothiazide
- hydrocodone bitartrate
- hydrocodone polistirex
- hydrocortis valerate
- hydrocortisone
- Hydrocortone
- Hydro-D
- HydroDIURIL
- hydroflumethiazide
- hydrogen peroxide
- Hydromax
- Hydromet
- hydromorphone
- Hydropane syrup
- Hydropres
- hydroquinone
- hydroxocobalamin
- hydroxocoralamin
- hydroxychloroquine
- Hydroxycut
- hydroxypropyl
- hydroxyurea
- hydroxyzine pamoate
- Hygroton
- Hylaform
- Hylan GF
- Hylenex
- Hylorel
- hyoscine
- hyoscyamine
- Hypaque
- Hypaque
- Hypaque-Cysto
- Hypaquemeglumine
- Hyperab

## H

- ❏ HyperHep
- ❏ hypericum
- ❏ Hyperstat
- ❏ Hyper-Tet
- ❏ HypRho-D
- ❏ Hyrexin-50
- ❏ hypromellose
- ❏ Hyskon
- ❏ Hytakerol
- ❏ Hytone
- ❏ Hytrin
- ❏ Hyzaar

## I

- ❏ Iamin
- ❏ ibandronate
- ❏ Iberet-Folic
- ❏ ibritumomab tiuxetan
- ❏ IBU
- ❏ ibuprofen
- ❏ ibuprofen lysine
- ❏ Ibu-Tab
- ❏ Ibutilide
- ❏ IC-Green
- ❏ ichthammol
- ❏ Icy Hot
- ❏ Idamycin
- ❏ idarubicin
- ❏ Identi-Dose
- ❏ idoxuride
- ❏ idursulfase
- ❏ IFEX
- ❏ IFN-Alpha 2
- ❏ Ifosamide
- ❏ Iletin II, Lente
- ❏ Iletin II, NPH
- ❏ Ilopan
- ❏ Ilosone
- ❏ Ilotycin
- ❏ ILX B-12

## I

- ❏ Imagent
- ❏ imatinib mesylate
- ❏ Imdur
- ❏ Imferon
- ❏ imidazole
- ❏ imiglucerase
- ❏ imipenem
- ❏ imipenem & cilastatin
- ❏ imipramine pamoate
- ❏ imiquimod
- ❏ Imitrex
- ❏ Imivacurium
- ❏ ImmuGo
- ❏ Immulite
- ❏ Immunocal
- ❏ ImmunoLin
- ❏ Immunopro RX
- ❏ Imodium
- ❏ Imodium A-D
- ❏ Imogam
- ❏ Imovax
- ❏ Implanon
- ❏ ImpoAid
- ❏ Impregon
- ❏ Imuran
- ❏ Inapsine
- ❏ Increlex
- ❏ indapamide
- ❏ Inderal
- ❏ Inderide
- ❏ Indermil
- ❏ indinavir
- ❏ Indiplon
- ❏ Indium
- ❏ Indocid
- ❏ Indocin
- ❏ indocyanine green
- ❏ indomethacin
- ❏ Infanrix
- ❏ Infasurf
- ❏ InFeD

## I

- ❏ Infergen Singleject
- ❏ Inflamase
- ❏ infliximab
- ❏ influenza
- ❏ Infufer
- ❏ Infumorph
- ❏ Infuvite
- ❏ Innofem
- ❏ Innohep
- ❏ Innopran XL
- ❏ Innovar
- ❏ Inocor
- ❏ INOmax
- ❏ inositol
- ❏ INS365
- ❏ Inspra
- ❏ Insulatard
- ❏ insulin
- ❏ insulin aspart protamine
- ❏ insulin detemir
- ❏ insulin glargine
- ❏ insulin glulisine
- ❏ insulin human
- ❏ insulin lispro
- ❏ insulin lispro protamine
- ❏ Intal
- ❏ Integrilin
- ❏ Integrase inhibitors
- ❏ Intelectol
- ❏ Intelence
- ❏ Intensol
- ❏ Interceed [TC7]
- ❏ Interex
- ❏ interferon Alfa-2A
- ❏ interferon Alfa-2b
- ❏ interferon Alfacon
- ❏ interferon Alfa-N3
- ❏ interferon Beta-1A
- ❏ interferon Beta-1B
- ❏ interferon Gamma-1B
- ❏ Intergel

## I

- ❏ Interleukin-1
- ❏ Intimex
- ❏ Inti-Mist
- ❏ IntraCoil
- ❏ Intralipid 10 %
- ❏ Intrinsa patch
- ❏ Intron
- ❏ Intropaque
- ❏ Intropin
- ❏ inulin
- ❏ Invanz
- ❏ Invega
- ❏ Inversine
- ❏ Invirase
- ❏ iobenguane
- ❏ Ioxalan
- ❏ iodine
- ❏ iodoquinol
- ❏ iodoquinol
- ❏ iohexol
- ❏ Ionamin
- ❏ Ionil-T
- ❏ Ionsys transdermal
- ❏ Iontophoretic
- ❏ iopamidol
- ❏ iopanoic acid
- ❏ Iophen
- ❏ Iophylline
- ❏ iopidine
- ❏ iothalamate meglumine
- ❏ iothalamic acid
- ❏ ipecac
- ❏ iPlex
- ❏ IPOL vaccine
- ❏ ipratropium bromide
- ❏ ipriflavone
- ❏ Iprivask
- ❏ Ipsatol
- ❏ Iquix
- ❏ irbesartan
- ❏ Ircon
- ❏ Iressa

## I

- ❏ Irigate
- ❏ irinotecan
- ❏ Iromin-G
- ❏ iron
- ❏ iron carbonyl
- ❏ iron dextran
- ❏ iron polysaccharide
- ❏ iron sucrose
- ❏ Irospan
- ❏ Isatori Lean
- ❏ Iscar Quercus
- ❏ ISDN
- ❏ Isentress
- ❏ Ismelin
- ❏ Ismo
- ❏ isocarboxazid
- ❏ Isoclor
- ❏ isoetharine
- ❏ isoflurane
- ❏ isoflurophate
- ❏ isometheptene mucate
- ❏ isoniazid
- ❏ isoproterenol
- ❏ Isoptin SR
- ❏ Isopto Carbachol
- ❏ Isopto Carpine
- ❏ Isopto Eserine
- ❏ Isordil
- ❏ isosorbide
- ❏ isosorbide dinitrate
- ❏ isosorbide mononitrate
- ❏ isotretinoin
- ❏ Isoxsuprine
- ❏ Isovex
- ❏ Isovorin
- ❏ Isovue-128
- ❏ Isovue-200
- ❏ Isovue-300
- ❏ isoxsuprine
- ❏ isradipine
- ❏ Istalol

## I

- ❏ Isuprel
- ❏ Itch-X
- ❏ itraconazole
- ❏ Ivarest
- ❏ Iveegam
- ❏ ivermectin
- ❏ Ivy-Dry
- ❏ IvyStat!
- ❏ ixabepilone
- ❏ Ixempra

## J

- ❏ Jadelle
- ❏ Jantoven
- ❏ Janumet
- ❏ Januvia
- ❏ Jenest
- ❏ Je-Vax
- ❏ Jevity-Isotonic liquid
- ❏ Joint-Ritis
- ❏ Jolivette
- ❏ Junel
- ❏ Juvederm

## K

- ❏ Kabikinase
- ❏ Kadian
- ❏ Kaletra
- ❏ Kanamycin
- ❏ Kank-A
- ❏ Kantrex
- ❏ Kaoelectrolyte
- ❏ Kaopectate
- ❏ Kapectolin
- ❏ Kariva
- ❏ Karno Life
- ❏ Kava Kava
- ❏ Kayexalate

## K

- ❏ K-Dur microburst
- ❏ Keflex
- ❏ Keftab
- ❏ Kefurox
- ❏ Kefzol
- ❏ Kemadrin
- ❏ Kemstro
- ❏ Kenacort
- ❏ Kenalog
- ❏ Kepivance
- ❏ Keppra
- ❏ Keri Lotion
- ❏ Kerlone
- ❏ Ketalar
- ❏ Ketamine
- ❏ Ketek
- ❏ ketoconazole
- ❏ ketoprofen
- ❏ ketorolac tromethamine
- ❏ ketotifen
- ❏ Key-Pred SP
- ❏ Kidrolase
- ❏ Kie Syrup
- ❏ Kinerase
- ❏ Kineret
- ❏ Kinevac
- ❏ Kinrix
- ❏ Kionex
- ❏ Klaron
- ❏ Klondremul
- ❏ Klonopin
- ❏ K-Lor
- ❏ Klor-Con
- ❏ Klotrix
- ❏ Kneerelief
- ❏ Koate-DVI
- ❏ Koate-HP
- ❏ Kogenate
- ❏ KOH solution
- ❏ Kolantyl
- ❏ Kondremul

## K

- ❏ Konsyl
- ❏ Konyne
- ❏ Koo Sar
- ❏ Koro-Flex
- ❏ Koromex
- ❏ KP Duty
- ❏ K-Phos
- ❏ Kristalose
- ❏ Kronofed
- ❏ K-Tab
- ❏ Kudrox
- ❏ kunecatechins
- ❏ Kutrase
- ❏ Kuvan
- ❏ Ku-Zyme
- ❏ Kwell
- ❏ KY-Plus
- ❏ Kytril

## L

- ❏ L-arginine
- ❏ L-gluatmic acid
- ❏ L-gluatmine
- ❏ labetalol
- ❏ Lac-Hydrin
- ❏ Laclotion
- ❏ lacosamide
- ❏ Lacri-Lube
- ❏ Lacrisert
- ❏ LactAid
- ❏ lactalbumin hydrolysate
- ❏ lactase
- ❏ lactic acid
- ❏ Lacticare
- ❏ Lactinol
- ❏ lactobacillus reuteri
- ❏ Lactocal
- ❏ lactulose
- ❏ Lamictal
- ❏ Lamisil

## L

- ☐ Lamisil/Terbinafine
- ☐ lamivudine
- ☐ lamotrigine
- ☐ Lamprene
- ☐ lamotrigine
- ☐ Lanacane
- ☐ lanolin
- ☐ Lanophyllin
- ☐ Lanoxicaps
- ☐ Lanoxin
- ☐ lanreotide acetate
- ☐ lansoprazole
- ☐ lanthanum carbonate
- ☐ Lantus
- ☐ Lantus SoloStar
- ☐ lapatinib
- ☐ Lariam
- ☐ Laradopa
- ☐ Largactil
- ☐ laronidase
- ☐ Lasix
- ☐ Latanoprost
- ☐ Latisse
- ☐ Laudanum
- ☐ Lazerformaldehyde
- ☐ Lazersporin
- ☐ L-Carnitine
- ☐ Lecithin
- ☐ L-Cystine
- ☐ Ledercillin
- ☐ Leena
- ☐ leflunomide
- ☐ Legatrin
- ☐ lenalidomide
- ☐ Lente Iletin
- ☐ lepirudin
- ☐ Leptoprin
- ☐ lercanidipine
- ☐ Lescol
- ☐ Lessina
- ☐ Letairis

## L

- ☐ letrozole
- ☐ Leucovorin
- ☐ Leucovorin rescue
- ☐ Leukeran
- ☐ Leukine
- ☐ Leukotriene
- ☐ leuprolide
- ☐ Leustatin
- ☐ levalbuterol
- ☐ levamisole
- ☐ levallorphan
- ☐ Levaquin
- ☐ Levatol
- ☐ Levbid
- ☐ Levemir
- ☐ levetiracetam
- ☐ Levitra
- ☐ Levlen
- ☐ Levlite
- ☐ levmetamfetamine
- ☐ levobetaxolol
- ☐ levobunolol
- ☐ levobupivacaine
- ☐ levocabastine
- ☐ levocarnitine
- ☐ levocetirizine dihydrochloride
- ☐ levodopa
- ☐ Levo-Dromoran
- ☐ levofloxacin
- ☐ Levolet
- ☐ Levoleucovorin
- ☐ levomethadyl acetate
- ☐ levonorgestrel
- ☐ Levoprome
- ☐ Levoquin
- ☐ Levora
- ☐ Levo-T
- ☐ levorphanol
- ☐ Levothroid
- ☐ levothyroxine
- ☐ Levoxyl

| **L** | **L** |
|---|---|

- ❑ Levsin
- ❑ Levsinex Timecaps
- ❑ Levulan Kerastick
- ❑ Lexapro
- ❑ Lexidronam
- ❑ Lexiscan
- ❑ Lexiva
- ❑ Lexxel
- ❑ Lialda
- ❑ Libra
- ❑ Librax
- ❑ Libritabs
- ❑ Librium
- ❑ Lidex
- ❑ lidocaine
- ❑ Lidoderm patch
- ❑ lidoflazine
- ❑ LidoPen Auto-Injector
- ❑ LidoSite
- ❑ Lifegenes spray
- ❑ Lifepak capsules
- ❑ Limbitrol
- ❑ Limbrel
- ❑ Lincocin
- ❑ Lincomycin
- ❑ Lindane
- ❑ Linezolid
- ❑ Linosamide
- ❑ Lioresal
- ❑ liothyronine
- ❑ Liotrix
- ❑ Lipase
- ❑ Lipitor
- ❑ lipoic acid
- ❑ Liposyn 10 %
- ❑ LipoTrim
- ❑ Liquibid
- ❑ Liqui-Char
- ❑ Liquipake
- ❑ Liquipred
- ❑ Liquiprin

- ❑ lisdexamfetamine dimesylate
- ❑ lisinopril
- ❑ lithium carbonate
- ❑ lithium citrate
- ❑ Lithobid
- ❑ Lithonate
- ❑ Lithostat
- ❑ Lithotabs
- ❑ Little Tummys
- ❑ Livial
- ❑ Lixolin
- ❑ L.M.X.4 cream
- ❑ L.M.X.5 cream
- ❑ LMD 10 %
- ❑ L-O-M Mus softgel
- ❑ LoCholest
- ❑ Locoid Lipocreme
- ❑ Lodine
- ❑ Lodosyn
- ❑ Lodox
- ❑ Lodoxamide
- ❑ Lodoxide
- ❑ Lodrane
- ❑ Loestrin
- ❑ Loestrin 24 Fe
- ❑ Lofibra
- ❑ lomefloxacin
- ❑ Lomotil
- ❑ lomustine
- ❑ Loniten
- ❑ Lonox
- ❑ Lo/Ovral
- ❑ loperamide
- ❑ Lopid
- ❑ lopinavir
- ❑ Lopressor
- ❑ Loprox
- ❑ Lorabid
- ❑ loracarbef
- ❑ loratadine
- ❑ lorazepam

## L

- ❏ Lorcet
- ❏ L'Oreal
- ❏ Lorelco
- ❏ Lorfan
- ❏ Loridine
- ❏ Lortab
- ❏ losartan
- ❏ LoSeasonique
- ❏ Lotemax
- ❏ Lotensin
- ❏ loteprednol
- ❏ Lotrel
- ❏ Lotrimin
- ❏ Lotrisone
- ❏ Lotrix
- ❏ Lotronex
- ❏ Lovaza
- ❏ Lovpil
- ❏ Low-Ogestrel
- ❏ lovastatin
- ❏ Lovenox
- ❏ Loxapine
- ❏ Loxitane
- ❏ Lozol
- ❏ LSAID
- ❏ LSD
- ❏ lubiprostone
- ❏ Lubriderm
- ❏ Lubrin
- ❏ Lucentis
- ❏ Ludiomil
- ❏ Lufyllin-GG
- ❏ Lumigan
- ❏ Lunelle
- ❏ Lunesta
- ❏ Lupron
- ❏ Luride
- ❏ Lurline
- ❏ Lusedra
- ❏ Lustra
- ❏ lutein

## L

- ❏ Lutera
- ❏ Lutrepulse
- ❏ lutropin alfa
- ❏ Luveris
- ❏ Luvox
- ❏ Luxiq foam
- ❏ Lybrel
- ❏ lycopene
- ❏ LYMErix
- ❏ Lymphazurin
- ❏ Lypressin
- ❏ Lyrica
- ❏ lysergic acid diethylamide
- ❏ Lysine
- ❏ Lysodren

## M

- ❏ MAA kit
- ❏ Maalox
- ❏ Macrobid
- ❏ Macrodantin
- ❏ macrolide
- ❏ Macugen
- ❏ Macutein
- ❏ mafenide acetate
- ❏ Mag-al
- ❏ Magan
- ❏ Ma Huang
- ❏ Magnaril
- ❏ magnesium
- ❏ magnesium carbonate
- ❏ magnesium hydroxide
- ❏ magnesium oxide
- ❏ magnesium sulfate
- ❏ magnesium trisilicate
- ❏ Magnevist
- ❏ Magnolax
- ❏ Magonate
- ❏ Mag-Ox
- ❏ Magsal

## M

- Magtab SR
- Maintain
- Malarone
- Malathion
- Maltsupex
- Mandelamine
- ManDelay
- Mandol
- Manerex
- Mangafodipir
- manganese
- Mann-Dino
- Mannitol
- Mantadil
- MAO inhibitor
- Maox
- maprotiline
- maraviroc
- Marax
- Marblen
- Marcaine
- MarineOmega
- Marinol
- Marlyn
- Marplan
- Marvelon
- Massengill douche
- Masoprocol
- Materna
- Matulane
- Mavik
- Maxair Autohaler
- Maxalt
- Maxalt-MLT
- Maxaquin
- Maxidex
- Maxidone
- Maxifed
- Maxiflor
- Maxipime
- Maxitrol

## M

- Maxzide
- May-Vita
- Mazepine
- mazindo
- MDP Kit
- MDR Fitness
- Mebaral
- mebendazole
- mecamylamine
- mecasermin
- mechlorethamine
- Meclan
- meclizine
- meclofenamate
- Meclomen
- Mederma
- Medifast
- Medigesic
- Mediplex
- Medizym
- Medi-Zyme
- Medrol
- medroxyprogesterone
- mefenamic acid
- mefloquine
- Mefoxin
- Mega-B
- Megace
- Megadose
- Mega MSM
- megestrol acetate
- Melanex
- melatonin
- Mellaril
- meloxicam
- melphalan
- MEM 1414
- memantine
- Menactra
- Menest
- Menocheck

## M

- ❑ Menomune
- ❑ Menostar
- ❑ menotropin
- ❑ Mentax
- ❑ mepenzolate bromide
- ❑ Mepergan
- ❑ meperidine
- ❑ mephobarbital
- ❑ Mephyton
- ❑ mepivacaine
- ❑ meprobamate
- ❑ Mepron
- ❑ Mequinol
- ❑ mercaptopurine
- ❑ Merci Retreiver
- ❑ Mercurochrome
- ❑ Meribin
- ❑ Meridia
- ❑ meropenem
- ❑ Merrem I.V.
- ❑ Mertazapine
- ❑ Merthiolate
- ❑ Meruvax
- ❑ mesalamine
- ❑ mesantoin
- ❑ Mescolor
- ❑ Mesna
- ❑ Mesnex
- ❑ mesoridazine
- ❑ Mestinon
- ❑ Mestranol
- ❑ Metab-O-Fx
- ❑ Metabolife
- ❑ Metadate-CD
- ❑ Metaglip
- ❑ Metahydrin
- ❑ Metamucil
- ❑ metaproterenol
- ❑ metaraminol bitartrate
- ❑ Metastron
- ❑ metaxalone

## M

- ❑ metformin
- ❑ methacholine
- ❑ methadone
- ❑ Methadose
- ❑ methamphetamine
- ❑ methaqualone
- ❑ methazolamide
- ❑ methenamine hippurate
- ❑ methimazole
- ❑ methionine
- ❑ methobarbital
- ❑ methocarbamol
- ❑ methohexital
- ❑ Methosalen
- ❑ methotrexate
- ❑ methoxamine
- ❑ methoxsalen
- ❑ methoxy polyethylene glycol-epoetin
- ❑ methscopolamine
- ❑ methsuximide
- ❑ methulose
- ❑ methyclothiazide
- ❑ methyl aminolevulinate
- ❑ methylatropine bromide
- ❑ methyldopa
- ❑ methyldopate
- ❑ methylene blue
- ❑ methylene trichloride
- ❑ methylergonovine
- ❑ methyl green
- ❑ Methylin
- ❑ methylnaltrexone bromide
- ❑ methylphenidate
- ❑ methylpred
- ❑ methylprednisolone
- ❑ methyl salicylate
- ❑ methyl sulfate
- ❑ methyltestosterone
- ❑ methylthiouracil
- ❑ methyl violet
- ❑ methyl xanthine

| M | M |
|---|---|
| ❑ methysergide | ❑ midodrine |
| ❑ Metimyd | ❑ Midol |
| ❑ metoclopramide | ❑ Midrin |
| ❑ metocurine iodide | ❑ Miveprev |
| ❑ metolazone | ❑ Mifeprex |
| ❑ metoprolol succinate | ❑ mifepristone [RU486] |
| ❑ metoprolol tartrate | ❑ Miglitol |
| ❑ MetroCream | ❑ miglustat |
| ❑ Metrodin | ❑ MigraHealth |
| ❑ MetroGel | ❑ Migra Migraine spray |
| ❑ MetroLotion | ❑ Migralam |
| ❑ metronidazole | ❑ Migranal |
| ❑ metropirone | ❑ Milk of Magnesia |
| ❑ Metubine | ❑ Milkinol |
| ❑ Metvixia | ❑ milnacipran |
| ❑ metyrapone | ❑ Milontin |
| ❑ metyrosine | ❑ Milophene |
| ❑ Mevacor | ❑ milrinone |
| ❑ mevastatin | ❑ Miltown |
| ❑ mexiletine | ❑ Mimyx cream |
| ❑ Mexitil | ❑ minerals |
| ❑ Mezlin | ❑ mineral oil |
| ❑ mezlocillin | ❑ Minestrin |
| ❑ MHP TakeOff Hi-Energy | ❑ Minipress |
| ❑ micafungin | ❑ Minitran |
| ❑ Miacalcin | ❑ Minit-Rub |
| ❑ Micanol | ❑ Minitran |
| ❑ Micardis | ❑ Minizide |
| ❑ Micatin | ❑ Minocin |
| ❑ miconazole | ❑ minocycline |
| ❑ Micort-HC | ❑ minoxidil |
| ❑ MICRhoGAM | ❑ Mintezole |
| ❑ Micro-K | ❑ Miocel |
| ❑ Microgestin | ❑ Miochol |
| ❑ Microgestin Fe | ❑ Mio-Rel |
| ❑ Micronase | ❑ Miostat |
| ❑ micronized colestipol | ❑ Miracle of Aloe Miracure |
| ❑ Micronor | ❑ Miradon |
| ❑ Microzide | ❑ MiraLAX |
| ❑ Midamor | ❑ Mirapex |
| ❑ Midazolam | ❑ Mircera |

## M

- Mircette
- Mirena
- mirtazapine
- misoprostol
- Mithracin
- mithramycin
- mitomycin
- mitotane
- mitoxantrone
- Mitozytrex
- MitraFlex
- Mivacron
- mivacurium
- Mixtard
- M-M-R II
- Moban
- Mobic
- Mobigesic
- Modafinil
- Modane
- Moderil
- ModiCon
- Modrastane
- Moduretic
- moexipril
- Moi-Stir
- Moisturel
- molindone
- mometasone furoate
- mometasone furoate monohydrate
- Monarc-M
- monascus purpuerus went
- Monistat
- monoamine oxidase inhibitor
- monobenzone
- Monocal
- Monocid
- Monoclate-P
- Monodox
- monofluorophosphate
- Monogesic

## M

- monohydrate
- Monoket
- Mononessa
- Mononine
- Monopril
- Mono-Vacc
- montelukast
- Monurol
- moricizine
- MOPP
- morphine sulfate
- morrhuate sodium
- Motofen
- Motrin
- MoviPrep
- Moxatag
- moxifloxacin
- Moxilin
- Mozobil
- M-R VAX
- MS-325
- MS Contin
- MSIR
- MSM
- MSTA
- MT100
- MTS
- Mucinex
- Mucinex Mini-Melts
- Muco-Fen
- Mucomyst
- Mucosil
- Mudrane
- Mumpsvax
- mupirocin
- Murine eye products
- Muro Gonio-Gel
- muromonab-CD3
- MUSE
- Mustargen
- Mutamycin

## M

- ❑ M.V.I.
- ❑ Myambutol
- ❑ Mycamine
- ❑ Mycelex
- ❑ Myclo
- ❑ Mycobutin
- ❑ Mycocide
- ❑ Mycolog
- ❑ mycophenolate mofetil
- ❑ mycophenolic
- ❑ Mycostatin
- ❑ Myerlan
- ❑ Myfortic
- ❑ Mykrox
- ❑ Mylanta
- ❑ Myleran
- ❑ Mylicon
- ❑ Mylotarg
- ❑ Myobloc
- ❑ myochrysine
- ❑ Myoflex
- ❑ Myoview
- ❑ Myozyme
- ❑ myrrh
- ❑ Mysoline
- ❑ Mytelase
- ❑ Mytozytrex
- ❑ Mytrate
- ❑ Mytrex
- ❑ M-Zole 3

## N

- ❑ NABI-HB
- ❑ nabilone
- ❑ nabumetone
- ❑ nadolol
- ❑ Nadopen
- ❑ Nadostine
- ❑ Nafarelin
- ❑ Naftin

## N

- ❑ nalbuphine
- ❑ nafcillin
- ❑ naftifine
- ❑ Naftin
- ❑ Naglazyme
- ❑ nalbuphine
- ❑ Nalex
- ❑ Nalfon
- ❑ nalidixic acid
- ❑ Nallpen
- ❑ nalmefene
- ❑ naloxone
- ❑ naltrexone
- ❑ Namenda
- ❑ nambutone
- ❑ nandrolone decanoate
- ❑ naphazoline
- ❑ Naphcon A
- ❑ Naprelan
- ❑ Naprosyn
- ❑ naproxen
- ❑ naproxen sodium
- ❑ Naqua
- ❑ naratriptan
- ❑ Narcan
- ❑ Nardil
- ❑ Naropin
- ❑ Nasacort AQ
- ❑ NasalCrom
- ❑ Nasalide
- ❑ Nasarel
- ❑ Nasatab
- ❑ Nascobal
- ❑ Nasonex
- ❑ Natachew
- ❑ Natafort
- ❑ natalizumab
- ❑ natamycin
- ❑ nateglinide
- ❑ Natrecor
- ❑ Natrol

| N | N |
|---|---|

- ❏ Natrol CitriMax
- ❏ Nature's Bounty Xtreme Lean
- ❏ Nature-throid
- ❏ Naturetin
- ❏ Nauzene
- ❏ Navane
- ❏ Navelbine
- ❏ Navstel
- ❏ Nebcin
- ❏ nebivolol
- ❏ NebuPent
- ❏ Necon
- ❏ nedocromil
- ❏ N.E.E.
- ❏ nefazodone
- ❏ NegGram
- ❏ nelarabine
- ❏ nelfinavir
- ❏ Nelfon
- ❏ Nelova
- ❏ Nelulen
- ❏ Nembutal
- ❏ Neo-Codema
- ❏ Neo-Cortef
- ❏ Neo-Decadron
- ❏ Neo-Delta-Cortef
- ❏ Neolax
- ❏ Neoloid
- ❏ Neo-Medrol
- ❏ neomycin
- ❏ Neo-Polycin
- ❏ NeoProfen
- ❏ Neoral
- ❏ Neosar
- ❏ Neosporin
- ❏ neostigmine
- ❏ Neo-Synephrine
- ❏ NeoTect
- ❏ Neothylline
- ❏ Neovastat
- ❏ Neozin

- ❏ nepafenac
- ❏ NephrAmine
- ❏ Nephro-Calci
- ❏ Nephrocaps
- ❏ Nephro-Fer
- ❏ Nephro-Vite Rx
- ❏ Nephrox
- ❏ Neptazane
- ❏ Nesacaine
- ❏ nesiritide
- ❏ Nestabs CBF
- ❏ netilmicin
- ❏ Netromycin
- ❏ Neulasta
- ❏ Neumega
- ❏ Neupogen
- ❏ Neupro
- ❏ Neuro-Balance
- ❏ Neuromag
- ❏ Neuromins-DHA
- ❏ Neurontin
- ❏ Neutrexin
- ❏ Neutrogena
- ❏ Nevanac
- ❏ nevirapine
- ❏ Nexavar
- ❏ Nexium
- ❏ Nexterone
- ❏ Niacin
- ❏ niacinamide
- ❏ Niacor
- ❏ Niaspan
- ❏ nicardipine
- ❏ NicoDerm CQ
- ❏ Nicolar
- ❏ Nicomide
- ❏ Nicorette gum
- ❏ Nicosyn
- ❏ Nicotinamide
- ❏ nicotine polacrilex
- ❏ Nicotinex

## N

- ❑ nicotinic acid
- ❑ Nicotrol
- ❑ nifedipine
- ❑ Niferex
- ❑ Nilandron
- ❑ nilotinib
- ❑ Nilstat
- ❑ nilutamide
- ❑ Nimbex
- ❑ nimodipine
- ❑ Nimotop
- ❑ Niox
- ❑ Nipent
- ❑ Niravam
- ❑ nisoldipine
- ❑ nitazoxanide
- ❑ nitisinone
- ❑ Nitrek
- ❑ Nitro-Bid
- ❑ Nitrodisc
- ❑ Nitro-Dur
- ❑ nitrofurantoin
- ❑ nitrofurazone
- ❑ nitroglycerin
- ❑ Nitrol
- ❑ Nitrolingual Pumpspray
- ❑ NitroMist
- ❑ Nitrostat
- ❑ nitrous oxide
- ❑ Nix Shampoo
- ❑ nizatidine
- ❑ Nizoral A-D
- ❑ NoDoz
- ❑ Nolahist
- ❑ Nolamine
- ❑ Nolvadex
- ❑ nonoxynol-9
- ❑ Nora-BE
- ❑ Norcept
- ❑ Norco
- ❑ Norcuron

## N

- ❑ Nordette
- ❑ Norditropin
- ❑ Norel DM
- ❑ Norel SR
- ❑ norelgestromin
- ❑ norethindrone
- ❑ Norflex
- ❑ norfloxacin
- ❑ Norgesic
- ❑ norgestimate
- ❑ norgestrel
- ❑ Norinyl
- ❑ Noritate
- ❑ Norlestrin
- ❑ Normiflo
- ❑ Normodyne
- ❑ Noroxin
- ❑ Norpace
- ❑ Norplant
- ❑ Norpramin
- ❑ Nor-QD
- ❑ Nortemp
- ❑ Nortrel
- ❑ nortriptyline
- ❑ Norvasc
- ❑ Norvir
- ❑ Novacet
- ❑ Novaldex
- ❑ Novamine
- ❑ Novamoxin
- ❑ Novantrone
- ❑ Novarel
- ❑ Novitra
- ❑ Novocain
- ❑ Novolin
- ❑ NovoLog
- ❑ Novopen
- ❑ NovoSeven
- ❑ Novo-Thalidone
- ❑ Novothyrox
- ❑ novotriphyl

## N

- ❑ Noxafil
- ❑ Noxzema
- ❑ NPH Iletin
- ❑ Nplate
- ❑ NSAID
- ❑ NT-Kinase
- ❑ NU-Iron
- ❑ Nubain
- ❑ Nucofed
- ❑ NuFill
- ❑ Nuflexxa
- ❑ NuLev
- ❑ NuLYTLEY
- ❑ Numorphan
- ❑ Numzident
- ❑ Num-Zit-Gel
- ❑ Nunaturals LevelRight
- ❑ Nupercainal
- ❑ Nuromax
- ❑ Nutracort
- ❑ Nutropin
- ❑ Nutropin AQ
- ❑ Nutropin Nuspin
- ❑ Nutropin Pen
- ❑ NuvaRing
- ❑ Nuvigil
- ❑ Nuvion
- ❑ Nydrazid
- ❑ Nyquil
- ❑ Nystatin
- ❑ Nystop
- ❑ Nytilax
- ❑ Nytol

## O

- ❑ OBEGYN
- ❑ Obinex
- ❑ Oby-Cap
- ❑ OCC
- ❑ Ocean

## O

- ❑ Octagam
- ❑ octocrylene
- ❑ octoxynol-9
- ❑ octreotide acetate
- ❑ octyl dimethyl
- ❑ Ocu-Chlor
- ❑ Ocucoat
- ❑ Ocufen
- ❑ Ocuflox
- ❑ OcuFresh
- ❑ OcuHist
- ❑ Ocu-Mycin
- ❑ Ocusol
- ❑ Ocu-Spor
- ❑ Ocusporin
- ❑ Ocu-Sul
- ❑ Ocusulf
- ❑ Ocutricin
- ❑ ofloxacin
- ❑ OGEN
- ❑ Ogestrel
- ❑ OKA
- ❑ olanzapine
- ❑ Olay
- ❑ Olay Regenerist
- ❑ oleandomycin
- ❑ olive oil
- ❑ olmesartan medoxomil
- ❑ olopatadine
- ❑ olsalazine
- ❑ Olux Foam
- ❑ Olux-E Foam
- ❑ Omacor
- ❑ omalizumab
- ❑ omega-3 acids
- ❑ omega-3 ethyl esters
- ❑ omega-3 polyunsaturates
- ❑ omeprazole
- ❑ Omnaris
- ❑ Omnicef
- ❑ OmniHIB

**O**

- Omnihist
- Omnipaque
- Omnipen
- Omniscan
- Omnitrope
- Oncaspar
- Oncolym
- Oncovin
- ondansetron
- One-A-Day Weight Smart
- On-Q
- Ontak
- Ony-Clear
- Opana
- Opana ER
- Opcon-A
- Ophthacet
- Ophthaine
- Ophthetic
- Ophthochlor
- Ophthocort
- Ophtho-Diprivefrin
- oprelvekin
- Optaflu
- Opticrom
- OptiGold
- OptiMark
- Optimine
- Optimyd
- Optipranolol
- Optiray
- Optivar
- Optson
- Orabase
- Oracea
- OraDisc A
- Oragrafin
- Orajel
- Oramorph
- Orap
- Oraphen-PD

**O**

- Orapred
- Oraqix
- OraVerse
- OraVescent Fentanyl
- OrCel
- Orencia
- Oretic
- Orex
- Orfadin
- Organidin NR
- Orgaran
- Orinase
- Orlaam
- Orlistat
- Ornade
- Ornex
- orphenadrine
- orphengesic
- Ortho-Cept
- Orthoclone OKT3
- Ortho-Creme
- Ortho-Cyclen
- Ortho-Dienestrol
- Ortho-Est
- Ortho-Gynol
- Ortho Micronor
- Ortho-Novum
- Ortho-Prefest
- Ortho Evra
- Ortho Tri-Cyclen
- Ortho Tri-Cyclen Lo
- Orthovisc
- Orudis
- Oruvail
- Orzel
- Os-Cal
- Oscillo
- Oscillococcinum
- oseltamivir
- OsmoCyte
- Osmoglyn

## O

- OsmoPrep
- Osteo Bi-Flex
- Otocain
- OvaRex
- Ovcon
- Ovide
- Ovidrel
- Ovocyclin
- Ovral
- Ovrette
- Oxacillin
- Oxaine
- oxaliplatin
- Oxandrin
- oxandrolone
- oxaprozin
- Oxazepam
- oxazolidinone
- oxcarbazepine
- oxiconazole
- Oxilan
- Oxistat
- Oxsoralen
- oxtriphylline
- Oxy
- oxybenzone
- oxybutynin chloride
- oxycodone
- OxyContin
- OxyFast
- OxyIR
- oxymetazoline
- oxymetholone
- oxymorphone
- oxyquinoline
- Oxyspectro
- Oxystat
- oxytetracycline
- oxytocin
- Oxytrol
- Ozogamicin

## P

- PA-824
- Pacaps
- Pacerone
- paclitaxel
- Paddock Podofliox
- padimate
- Pain Bust
- PainPatch
- Palaron
- palifermin
- paliperidone
- palivizumab
- Palladone
- Palmatate
- palonosetron HCl
- pamabrom
- Pamelor
- pamidronate
- Pamine
- Pamprin
- Panafil
- Panafil SE
- Panalgesic Gold Cream
- Panax
- Pancrease MT
- pancreatin
- pancrelipase
- pancuronium bromide
- Pandel
- Panglobulin NF
- Panhematin
- panitumumab
- Panmycin
- PanOxyl
- Panretin
- Panthenol
- pantoprazole
- pantothenate calcium
- pantothenic acid
- Panwarfin
- papain

## P

- papaverine
- papillomavirus
- para-amino benzoic acid
- Paradione
- Paraflex
- Parafon Forte
- ParaGard T380 A
- paraldehyde
- Paraplatin
- Parathar
- paregoric
- Parcopa
- Paremyd
- parepectolin
- paricalcitol
- Parlodel
- Parnate
- paroxetine
- Paser
- Patady
- Patanase
- Patanol
- PatentLean
- Pathiam
- Pathocil
- Pavabid
- Pavulon
- Paxil
- Paxil CR
- Pazo
- PBZ
- PCE
- PCP
- PC Spes
- PDE5 blocker
- PediaCare
- Pediacof
- Pediaflor
- Pedia-Lax
- Pedialyte
- Pediapred

## P

- Pediarix
- PediaSure
- Pediazole
- Pedi-Boro Soak Paks
- Pedi-Dri
- PediOtic
- PedvaxHIB
- PEG-3350
- pegademase
- Peganone
- pegaptanib
- pegaspargase
- Pegasys
- pegfilgrastim
- PEG-Intron
- peginterferon Alfa-2B
- pegvisomant
- pemetrexed
- pemirolast
- Pemoline
- penbutolol
- Pen-Colate
- penciclovir
- Penecort
- Penetrex
- penicillin
- penicillin G benzathine
- pencicillin G procaine
- penicillamine
- Penlac
- Pentacel
- Pentam
- pentamidine
- Pentamycetin
- Pentasa
- Pentaspan
- Pentastarch
- pentazocine
- Pentetate
- pentobarbital
- pentosan polysulfate sodium

## P

- pentostatin
- Pentothal, Sodium
- pentoxifylline
- Pentoxil
- Pen-Vee
- Pep-Back
- Pepcid
- Pepcid AC
- Peptavlon
- peptidase
- Pepto-Bismol
- peptolide
- Perbuterol
- Percocet
- Percodan
- Percogesic
- Percolone
- Perdiem
- Perflutren lipid microspheres
- Perform
- Perforomist
- pergolide
- Pergonal
- Periactin
- Peri-Colace
- Peridex
- Peridin-C
- perindopril erbumine
- Periochip
- Periogard
- Periostat
- Perlane
- Permax
- permethrin
- perphenazine
- Persantine
- pethidine
- Pfizerpen
- Phazyme
- Phenaphen
- phenazopyridine

## P

- Phencyclidine
- phendimetrazine tartrate
- phenelzine
- Phenergan
- pheniramine
- Phenobarbital
- phenol
- phenolphthalein
- phenothiazine
- phenoxybenzamine
- phenserine
- phentermine
- phentolamine
- phenurone
- phenylalanine
- phenylazo-diamino-pyridine
- phenylephrine
- phenylprine
- phenylpropanolamine
- phenyl salicylate
- phenyltoloxamine
- Phenytek
- phenytoin
- Phillips Milk of Magnesia
- pHisoDerm
- pHisoHex
- Phoschol
- PhosLo
- phosphatidylcholine
- phosphodiesterase inhibitor
- phospholine iodide
- phosphomycin
- Photofrin
- Phrenilin Forte
- Phyllocontin
- physostigmine
- phytoene
- phytoestrogen
- phytofluene
- phytonadione
- Phytoplex

## P

- ❏ phytosterol blocker
- ❏ Phyto-Vite
- ❏ Picovir
- ❏ Pilocar
- ❏ pilocarpine
- ❏ Pilocel
- ❏ Pima
- ❏ pimecrolimus
- ❏ pimozide
- ❏ pindolol
- ❏ Pin-Rid
- ❏ pioglitazone
- ❏ Pipecuronium
- ❏ piperacillin
- ❏ Pipracil
- ❏ pirbuterol
- ❏ Pirfenidone
- ❏ piroxicam
- ❏ Pitocin
- ❏ Pitressin Synthetic
- ❏ PKC
- ❏ Placidyl
- ❏ Plan B
- ❏ plantago ovata
- ❏ Plaquenil
- ❏ PLAS+SD
- ❏ Plasbumin
- ❏ Plasma-Lyte
- ❏ Plasmanate
- ❏ Plasma-Plex
- ❏ plasma protein fraction
- ❏ Plasmatein
- ❏ Platinol-AQ
- ❏ Plavix
- ❏ Pleconaril
- ❏ Plegisol
- ❏ Plenaxis
- ❏ Plendil
- ❏ plerixafor
- ❏ Pletal
- ❏ Plexion

## P

- ❏ plicamycin
- ❏ PMS Theophylline
- ❏ Pneumomist
- ❏ Pneumotussin HC
- ❏ Pneumovax
- ❏ Pnu-Imune 23
- ❏ Podocon
- ❏ podofilox
- ❏ podophyllin
- ❏ polifeprosan 20
- ❏ polistirex
- ❏ Polocaine
- ❏ Polycitra
- ❏ polyethylene glycol
- ❏ Polygam S/D
- ❏ Polyhistine
- ❏ Polymox
- ❏ polymyxin
- ❏ polypeptide
- ❏ Polyphenon E
- ❏ polysaccharide iron
- ❏ Polyspectrin
- ❏ Polysporin
- ❏ Polytar shampoo
- ❏ polythiazide
- ❏ Polytrim
- ❏ polyurethane
- ❏ polyvinyl chloride
- ❏ Poly-Vi-Sol
- ❏ POMP
- ❏ Ponaris
- ❏ Ponstel
- ❏ Pontocaine
- ❏ Poractant Alfa
- ❏ porfimer sodium
- ❏ Portia
- ❏ posaconazole
- ❏ Posicor
- ❏ Potaba
- ❏ Potaba envules
- ❏ potassium bitartrate

## P

- ☐ potassium chloride
- ☐ potassium citrate
- ☐ povidone iodide
- ☐ pralidoxime chloride
- ☐ Pramasone
- ☐ Pramilet
- ☐ pramipexole
- ☐ pramlintide
- ☐ Pramosone
- ☐ pramoxine
- ☐ Pranactin
- ☐ PrandiMet
- ☐ Prandin
- ☐ Pravachol
- ☐ Pravagard
- ☐ pravastatin
- ☐ pravastin
- ☐ Prax
- ☐ praziquantel
- ☐ prazosin
- ☐ PreCare Prenatal
- ☐ Precedex
- ☐ Precose
- ☐ Pred Forte
- ☐ prednicarbate
- ☐ Prednicen
- ☐ prednisolone
- ☐ prednisone
- ☐ Prefrin
- ☐ Pregabalin
- ☐ Pregnyl
- ☐ Prelay
- ☐ Prelone
- ☐ Prelu-2
- ☐ Premarin
- ☐ PremesissRX
- ☐ Premphase
- ☐ Prempro
- ☐ Premsyn
- ☐ Prenate Ultra
- ☐ Preparation H

## P

- ☐ Prepcat
- ☐ Prepidil
- ☐ PreScrub
- ☐ Prestara
- ☐ Prevacid
- ☐ Prevalite
- ☐ Preven
- ☐ Prevident
- ☐ Prevnar
- ☐ Prevpac
- ☐ Prezista
- ☐ Prialt
- ☐ Prid
- ☐ Priftin
- ☐ prilocaine
- ☐ Prilosec
- ☐ Prilosec OTC
- ☐ Primacare
- ☐ Primacor
- ☐ primaquine
- ☐ Primatene mist
- ☐ Primaxin
- ☐ primidone
- ☐ Primsol
- ☐ Principen
- ☐ Prinivil
- ☐ Prinzide
- ☐ Primatene
- ☐ primidone
- ☐ Priscoline
- ☐ Pristiq
- ☐ Privigen
- ☐ ProAir HFA
- ☐ ProAmatine
- ☐ probenecid
- ☐ Probiata
- ☐ Probiotica
- ☐ Probucol
- ☐ procainamide
- ☐ ProcalAmine
- ☐ Procanbid

## P

- ❑ procarbazine
- ❑ Procardia
- ❑ Prochieve
- ❑ prochlorperazine
- ❑ Procleix
- ❑ Pro-Clerz
- ❑ Procosa II
- ❑ Procrit
- ❑ Proctocort
- ❑ Proctocream HC
- ❑ Proctofoam HC
- ❑ procyclidine
- ❑ Procylon
- ❑ Procytox
- ❑ Prodium
- ❑ Profasi
- ❑ Profen
- ❑ Profilnine SD
- ❑ Proflavanol
- ❑ Progesin
- ❑ Progestasert System
- ❑ progesterone
- ❑ Proglycem
- ❑ Prograf
- ❑ Prograniq
- ❑ proguanil
- ❑ ProHance
- ❑ ProHIBiT
- ❑ Prohim
- ❑ Prolab
- ❑ Prolastin
- ❑ Proleukin
- ❑ Prolex
- ❑ Prolixin
- ❑ Proloprim
- ❑ Promacta
- ❑ promazine
- ❑ Promensil
- ❑ Prometh
- ❑ promethazine
- ❑ Prometrium

## P

- ❑ Pronestyl
- ❑ pronutra protein
- ❑ Propade
- ❑ propafenone
- ❑ Propagest
- ❑ propantheline
- ❑ Proparacaine
- ❑ propatyl nitrate
- ❑ Propecia
- ❑ Prophyllin CCC
- ❑ propicillin
- ❑ Propine C Cap
- ❑ propiolactone
- ❑ Proplex T
- ❑ propofol
- ❑ propoxyphene
- ❑ propoxyphene napsylate
- ❑ propranolol
- ❑ Propulsid
- ❑ propyl alcohol
- ❑ propylene glycol
- ❑ propylhexedrine
- ❑ propylthiouracil
- ❑ Proquad
- ❑ Proquin XR
- ❑ Prosacea
- ❑ Proscar
- ❑ Prosed
- ❑ ProSol
- ❑ ProSom
- ❑ prostaglandin
- ❑ Prostaphlin
- ❑ Prostata
- ❑ ProStep
- ❑ Prostigmin
- ❑ Prostin
- ❑ Protamine sulfate
- ❑ Protamine zinc
- ❑ protease
- ❑ protease inhibitor
- ❑ Protenate

## P

- proteolytic enzyme
- Protex
- Protid
- protirelin
- proton pump inhibitor
- Protonix
- Protopam chloride
- Protophylline
- Protopic
- Protostat
- protriptyline
- Protropin
- Protuss
- Proventil
- Provera
- Provigil
- Provocholine
- Proxacol
- ProXtreme
- Prozac
- Prudoxin
- pseudoephedrine
- pseudoephedrine sulfate
- psoralens
- Psorcon
- Psoriasin gel
- psyllium
- PTK 787
- Pulexn DM
- Pumactant
- Pulmicort Flexhaler
- Pulmicort Respules
- Pulmicort Turbuhaler
- Pulmophylline
- Pulmozyme
- PureTrim
- Purinethol
- Pylera
- Pylori-Chek
- pyrantel pamoate
- pyrazinamide

## P

- Pyridium
- pyridostigmine
- pyridoxine
- pyrilamine
- pyrimethamine
- pyrithione

## Q

- Q-Bid
- Quaalude
- quadazocine
- quadrivalent
- Quadramet
- Quadrinal
- Quarzan
- Quanterra
- Quarzan
- Quasense
- Quelicin
- Questran
- quetiapine
- Quibron
- QuickClot
- quinacrine
- Quinaglute
- quinalan
- quinalbarbitone
- Quinaglute
- quinaldine blue
- Quinamm
- quinapril
- quinethazone
- Quinidex
- Quinidine
- Quinine
- quinolone
- quinupristin
- Quixin
- QVAR

| R |
|---|

- RabAvert
- rabeprazole
- Racivir
- Radiance injection
- Radiesse
- Radiogardase
- Ralivia
- raloxifene
- raltegravir
- ramelteon
- ramipril
- Ranexa
- ranibizumab
- ranitidine
- ranolazine
- rapacuronium
- Rapaflo
- Rapamune
- Rapinex
- Raplon
- Raptiva
- rasagiline mesylate
- rasburicase
- Rasilez
- Raxar
- Rauwolfia serpentina
- Rauzide
- Rayataz
- Razadyne
- RDH Bandage
- Reality
- Rebetol
- Rebetron
- Rebif
- Reclast
- Reclipsen
- Recombinant OspA
- Recombinate
- Recombivax
- Recothrom
- Redox

| R |
|---|

- Refacto
- Refludan
- regadenoson
- Regasporin
- Regitine
- Reglan
- Regonol
- Regranex
- Regroton
- Regulex
- Regutol
- Rehydralyte
- Reishimax
- Relafen
- Relagesic
- Releev
- Relenza
- Relistor
- Relpax
- Remeron
- REMERONSolTab
- Remicade
- remifentanil
- Reminyl
- Remodulin
- Remune
- Remular
- Renacidin irrigation
- Renagel
- RenAmin
- Renax
- Renedil
- Renese
- Renografin 60
- Reno-M-30
- Renova
- Renovue
- Renvela
- ReoPro
- repaglinide
- Replens

| R | R |
|---|---|

- Repronex
- RespiGam
- Requip
- Rescinnamine
- Rescon
- Rescriptor
- Rescula
- reserpine
- resorcinol
- Respa A.R.M.
- Respa-DM
- Respa-GF
- Respahist
- Respaire-SR
- Respbid
- RespiGam
- RESPeRATE
- Respihaler
- Respinol
- Resporal
- Restasis
- Restoril
- Restylane
- retapamulin
- Retavase
- Reteplase
- Retin-A
- Retisert
- Retrovir
- Revatio
- Reversol
- Revex
- ReVia
- Revimid
- Revlimid
- Rexata
- Reyataz
- Rezulin
- R-Gene 10
- Rheomacrodex
- Rheumatrex

- Rhinocort Aqua
- Rhinogesic
- Rhinosyn-X
- RhoGam
- Rhophylac
- Rhuli
- RhuMAb-E25
- ribasphere
- ribavirin
- riboflavin
- ricinoleic acid
- Ridaura
- Rid Mousse
- rifabutin
- Rifadin
- Rifamate
- rifampin
- rifapentine
- Rifater
- rifaximin
- rilonacept
- Rilutek
- riluzole
- Rimactane
- rimantadine
- rimonabant
- Rimso
- rinfabate
- Ringer's injection
- Ringer's lactated
- Riomet
- Riopan
- Riquent
- risedronate
- Risperdal
- risperidone
- Ritalin
- Ritodrine
- ritonavir
- Rituxan
- rituximab

## R

- rivastigmine
- rizatriptan
- RMS suppository
- Robaxin
- Robaxisal
- Robinul
- Robitussin
- Robitussin DAC
- Roc
- Rocaltrol
- Rocephin
- rocuronium bromide
- rofecoxib
- Roferon-A
- Rogaine
- Rogitine
- Rohto Zi
- Rohypnol
- Rolaids
- Rolaids softchews
- Romazicon
- romiplostim
- Rondec
- roofie
- ropinirole
- ropivacaine
- Rosac wash
- Rose Bengal
- Risets strips
- rosiglitazone
- rosuvastatin
- Rotahaler
- Rotarix
- RotaShield
- Rotateq
- rotavirus
- rotigotine
- Rowasa enema
- Roxanol
- Roxicet
- Roxicodone

## R

- Roxilox
- Roxiprin
- Rozerem
- RSV-IGIV
- RU-486 [mifepristone]
- Rubex
- rufinamide
- Rufludan
- Rum-K
- Rutoside
- Ryna-12
- Rynatan
- Rynatuss
- Rythmol
- Rythmol SR
- Ryzolt

## S

- sacosidase
- Safe-Tussin
- Saizen
- SalAc
- Sal-Acid plaster
- Salactic film
- Salagen
- Salflex
- salicylamide
- salicylic acid
- salicylsalicylic acid
- salmeterol xinafoate
- SangCya
- Salonpas
- Salonsip Aqua Patch
- Sal-Plant gel
- salsalate
- Saluron
- Salutensin
- SAM-e
- Sanctura
- Sanctura XR

## S

- Sancuso
- Sandimmune
- Sandoglobulin
- Sandostatin
- SangCya
- Sanorex
- Sansert
- Santyl
- sapropterin dihydrochloride
- saquinavir
- Sarafem
- Sarapin
- sargramostim
- Sativex
- Satogesic
- Savella
- Saw Palmetto
- SBR-Lipocream
- S-Caine Peel
- Scalpicin
- SCE-A
- Scleromate
- Sclerosol intrapleural
- scopolamine
- scopolamine hydrobromide
- Sculptra
- Seasonale
- Seasonique
- Sebazole
- Sebulex
- secobarbital
- Seconal
- SecreFlo
- Secretin
- Sectral
- Sedapap
- selegiline
- selenium
- selenium sulfide
- selenomethionine
- Selsun

## S

- Selzentry
- Semicid
- Semilente
- Semprex
- Sen Lo Fen
- senna
- sennosides
- Sen-Sei-Ro
- Senokot
- Senokotxtra
- Sensipar
- Sensorcaine
- Sepracor
- Septocaine
- Septra
- Ser-Ap-Es
- Serax
- Serentil
- Serevent
- sermorelin
- Seromycin
- Serophene
- Seroquel
- Serostim
- serotonin uptake inhibitor
- SERPACWA
- sertaconazole
- sertraline
- serum albumin
- Serutan
- Serzone
- sevelamer
- sevoflurane
- Sexativa Plus
- Sexelle
- shea butter
- shikonin
- Sibilium
- sibutramine
- sildenafil citrate
- Silmycin

## S

- ❑ silodosin
- ❑ Silvadene
- ❑ silver nitrate
- ❑ silver protein, mild
- ❑ silver sulfadiazine
- ❑ Simcor
- ❑ simethicone
- ❑ Similasan
- ❑ Simply Sleep
- ❑ Simulect
- ❑ simvastatin
- ❑ Sinarest
- ❑ Sincalide
- ❑ Sine-Aid
- ❑ Sinemet
- ❑ Sine-Aid
- ❑ Sine-Off
- ❑ Sinequan
- ❑ Sine-Relief
- ❑ Sinex
- ❑ Singulair
- ❑ SinoFresh
- ❑ Sinografin
- ❑ Sinulin
- ❑ Sinumist
- ❑ Sinutab
- ❑ Sinutuss
- ❑ Sinuvent
- ❑ sirolimus
- ❑ sitagliptin
- ❑ Skelaxin
- ❑ Skelid
- ❑ Sleep-eze
- ❑ Sleepinal
- ❑ Sleep-Max PM
- ❑ Sloan's liniment
- ❑ Slo-Bid
- ❑ Slo-Fe
- ❑ Slow-Mag
- ❑ Slo-Niacin
- ❑ Slo-Phyllin

## S

- ❑ SnoreStop
- ❑ SNO Strips
- ❑ sodium acid phosphate
- ❑ sodium benzoate
- ❑ sodium bicarbonate
- ❑ sodium brevital
- ❑ sodium chloride
- ❑ sodium citrate
- ❑ sodium diphosphate
- ❑ sodium ferric gluconate
- ❑ sodium fluoride
- ❑ sodium hyaluronate
- ❑ sodium oxybate
- ❑ sodium oxychlorosene
- ❑ sodium pentothal
- ❑ sodium phenylacetate
- ❑ sodium phosphate
- ❑ sodium propionate
- ❑ sodium sulamyd
- ❑ sodium sulfacetamide
- ❑ sodium sulfate
- ❑ Sojourn Sevoflurane
- ❑ Solage
- ❑ Solaquin
- ❑ Solaraze
- ❑ Solarcaine
- ❑ Solbar
- ❑ Solganal
- ❑ solifenacin succinate
- ❑ Soliris
- ❑ Solodyn
- ❑ Soltamox
- ❑ Solu-Cortef
- ❑ Solu-Medrol
- ❑ Solu-Phyllin
- ❑ Solurex
- ❑ Soma Compound
- ❑ SomatoKine
- ❑ somatostatin
- ❑ somatrem
- ❑ somatropin

| S | S |
|---|---|

- Somatuline Autogel
- Somatuline Depot
- Somavert
- Sominex
- Sonata
- SonoRX
- sorafenib
- sorbitol
- Sorbitrate
- Soriatane
- Sorine
- sotalol
- Sotradecol
- Sotret
- soy oil
- Spacer
- sparfloxacin
- Spectazole
- Spectracef
- Spectrobid
- Spenco 2$^{nd}$ Skin Scar
- spironolactone
- spiramycin
- Spiriva HandiHaler
- Sporanox
- Sportscreme
- Sprintek
- Sprycel
- Sronyx
- SSD cream
- SSD AF cream
- SSKI solution
- Stacker 2
- Stadol NS
- Stalevo
- Staminex
- Stanback
- stanozolol
- Starlix
- Staticin
- Statrol

- stavudine
- Stavzor
- Stelazine
- Sterapred
- Stilbestrol
- stilphostrol
- St. Ives
- St. John's Wort
- St. Joseph Aspirin
- Stopain
- Stoxil
- Strattera
- Streptase
- streptokinase
- Streptomycin
- streptozocin
- Striant
- Stridex
- StriVectin-HS
- StriVectin-SD
- Stromectol
- Strovite
- SU-101
- SU 11248
- Sublimaze
- Suboxone
- Subutex
- succimer
- succinylcholine
- succuss cineraria maritma
- Sucraid
- sucralfate
- Sucrets
- Sudafed
- Sufenta
- Sufentanil
- Sugen
- Sulamyd
- Sular
- sulbactam sodium
- sulfabenzamide

## S

- Sulfacet
- sulfacetamide sodium
- sulfadiazine
- sulfadoxine
- sulfamerazine
- sulfamethiazine
- sulfamethizole
- sulfamethoxazole
- Sulfamide
- Sulfamylon cream
- sulfanilamide
- SulfaPred
- sulfasalazine
- sulfinpyrazone
- sulfisoxazole
- sulfonamide
- Sulfonylurea
- Sulfoxyl
- sulfur
- sulindac
- Sultrin
- sumatriptan
- Sumycin
- sunitinib
- Sunril
- Supartz
- Super EPA
- Superfak
- superoxide dismutase
- Supprelin
- Supprelin LA
- Suprane
- Suprax
- Suprefact
- Sure Sleep
- Surfak
- Surmontil
- Surfak
- Survanta
- Sus-Phrine
- Sustaire

## S

- Sustiva
- Sutent
- Swabplus
- Swiss Kriss
- Syllact
- Symadine
- Symbicort
- Symbyax
- Symiotropin
- Symlin
- Symmetrel
- Symphasic
- Synagis
- Synalar
- Synalgos-DC
- Synarel
- Synemol
- Synera
- Synercid
- SynergyDefense
- Synophylate
- Synphasic
- Syprine
- Syn-Rx
- Synthroid
- Syntocinon
- Synvisc
- Syprine
- Systane

## T

- Tabloid
- TAC-3
- Taclonex
- tacrine
- tacrolimus
- tadalafil
- Tagamet
- Talacen
- Taclonex

| T | T |
|---|---|

- [ ] Talwin
- [ ] Tambocor
- [ ] Tamiflu
- [ ] tamoxifen
- [ ] tamsulosin
- [ ] Tanac
- [ ] Tanafed
- [ ] Tandem
- [ ] TAO
- [ ] Tapazole
- [ ] Tapentadol
- [ ] Tarceva
- [ ] Targretin
- [ ] Tarka
- [ ] Tasigna
- [ ] Tasmar
- [ ] Taurine
- [ ] Tavist D
- [ ] TAXUS Express 2
- [ ] Taxol
- [ ] Taxotere
- [ ] tazarotene
- [ ] Tazicef
- [ ] Tazidime
- [ ] tazobactam
- [ ] Tazorac
- [ ] Taztia
- [ ] TC7 [Interceed]
- [ ] TE Anatoxal Berna
- [ ] Teagreen
- [ ] Tears Naturale
- [ ] Tecnu
- [ ] Teczem
- [ ] tegaserod maleate
- [ ] Tegretol
- [ ] Tegison
- [ ] Tegopen
- [ ] Tegreen 97
- [ ] Tekturna
- [ ] Tekturna HCT
- [ ] Telbermin

- [ ] telbivudine
- [ ] Tel-E-Dose products
- [ ] Tel-E-Ject products
- [ ] Telepaque
- [ ] telithromycin
- [ ] telmesteine
- [ ] telmisartan
- [ ] Temaril
- [ ] temazepam
- [ ] Temodar
- [ ] Temovate
- [ ] temozolomide
- [ ] temsirolimus
- [ ] Tencon
- [ ] tenecteplase
- [ ] Tenex
- [ ] teniposide
- [ ] tenofovir disoproxil fumarate
- [ ] Tenoretic
- [ ] Tenormin
- [ ] Tensilon
- [ ] Tenuate
- [ ] Tequin
- [ ] Terazol
- [ ] terazosin
- [ ] terbinafine
- [ ] terbutaline
- [ ] terconazole
- [ ] Teril
- [ ] teriparatide
- [ ] terpin hydrate
- [ ] Terra-Cortril
- [ ] Terramycin
- [ ] Teslac
- [ ] Teslascan
- [ ] TESPA [TSPA]
- [ ] Tessalon
- [ ] Tessalon Perles
- [ ] Testerex
- [ ] Testim
- [ ] Testoderm TTS

| **T** | **T** |
|---|---|

- ❑ testolactone
- ❑ Testopel Pellet
- ❑ testosterone
- ❑ testosterone cypionate
- ❑ testosterone enanthate
- ❑ Testred
- ❑ tetrabenazine
- ❑ tetracaine
- ❑ tetracycline
- ❑ tetrahydrozoline
- ❑ Tetramune
- ❑ Tetrazene ES-50
- ❑ Teveten
- ❑ Teveten HCT
- ❑ Tev-Tropin
- ❑ Thalomid
- ❑ Thalidomide
- ❑ Thalitone
- ❑ Thalomid
- ❑ thallus chloride
- ❑ Tham
- ❑ Theo-24
- ❑ Theo-250
- ❑ Theo-Bid
- ❑ Theochron
- ❑ Theoclear
- ❑ Theocot
- ❑ Theo-dur
- ❑ Theolair
- ❑ Theomer
- ❑ theophylline
- ❑ theophylline anydrous
- ❑ Theostat
- ❑ Thiotepa
- ❑ Theo-Time
- ❑ Theovent
- ❑ Theo-X
- ❑ TheraCys
- ❑ Theradent
- ❑ TheraFlu
- ❑ Thera-Gesic

- ❑ Theramycin
- ❑ TheraPatch
- ❑ TheraTears
- ❑ ThermaCare
- ❑ Thermage
- ❑ ThermoDox
- ❑ Thermogenics
- ❑ thiabendazole
- ❑ thiamine
- ❑ thiamine disulfide
- ❑ thiazolidinedione
- ❑ thiethylperazine
- ❑ Thimerosal
- ❑ Thin-Patch
- ❑ ThinPrep
- ❑ Thinz
- ❑ thioguanine
- ❑ Thiola
- ❑ thiobarbiturates
- ❑ thiobutabarbital
- ❑ thiopental sodium
- ❑ Thioplex
- ❑ thioridazine
- ❑ thiotepa
- ❑ thiothixene
- ❑ Thonzonium
- ❑ Thorazine
- ❑ Thrombate III
- ❑ Thrombin-JMI
- ❑ Thylline
- ❑ Thymoglobulin
- ❑ Thymol
- ❑ thymus polypeptide
- ❑ Thyrel TRH
- ❑ Thyrogen
- ❑ thyroid
- ❑ Thyrolar
- ❑ ThyroSafe
- ❑ ThyroShield
- ❑ ThyroStart
- ❑ Thyro-Tab

## T

- Thyrotropin Alfa
- tiagabine
- Tiazac
- Tibolone
- Ticar
- ticarcillin
- TICE BCG
- Ticlid
- ticlopidine
- Tifacogin
- Tigan
- tigecycline
- Tikosyn
- Tilade Inhaler
- Tilia FE
- tiludronate
- Timentin
- Timolide
- timolol
- Timoptic
- Timoptic in ocudose
- Timoptic-XE
- Tinactin
- Tinamed
- Tindamax
- Tine test PPD
- Tineacide
- tinidazole
- tinzaparin
- tioconazole
- tiopronin
- tiotropium bromide
- tipranavir
- Tirofiban
- Tisseel VH fiber sealant
- Titralac
- tizanidine
- TNKase
- TOBI
- Tobradex
- tobramycin

## T

- Tobrex
- tocainide
- tocopheryl acetate
- Tofipan
- Tofipan-Z
- Tofranil
- Tolamide
- tolazamide
- tolazoline
- tolbutamide
- tolcapone
- Tolectin
- Tolinase
- tolmetin sodium
- Tolnaftate
- tolterodine
- Tomocat
- Tonocard
- Tonopaque
- Topamax
- Topicort
- topiramate
- topotecan
- Topricin
- Toprol XL
- Toradol
- torcetrapib
- Torecan
- toremifene
- Torisel
- Tornalate
- torsemide
- tositumomab
- Totect
- Totephan crème
- Toviaz
- TPA
- TPN electrolytes
- Tracleer
- Tracrium
- Tramadol

## T

- ❏ tranadik
- ❏ Trancopal
- ❏ Trandate
- ❏ trandolapril
- ❏ Transderm-Nitro patch
- ❏ Transderm SCOP patch
- ❏ Tranex
- ❏ tranexamic acid
- ❏ Tranxene
- ❏ Trastuzumab
- ❏ Trasylol
- ❏ TraumaDex Bandage
- ❏ Traumeel
- ❏ Travasol
- ❏ Travatan Z
- ❏ Travoprost
- ❏ trazodone
- ❏ Treanda
- ❏ Trecator-SC
- ❏ Trelstar Depot
- ❏ Trelstar LA
- ❏ Trental
- ❏ treprostinil sodium
- ❏ tretinoin
- ❏ Trexall
- ❏ Trexan
- ❏ Trexima
- ❏ Treximet
- ❏ Triactin
- ❏ triamcinolone
- ❏ Triam/HCTZ
- ❏ Triaminic
- ❏ Triaminic Softchews
- ❏ Triaminicin
- ❏ triamterene
- ❏ Tri-Sprintec
- ❏ Triavil
- ❏ Triaz
- ❏ triazolam
- ❏ tricarbocyanine
- ❏ trichlormethiazide

## T

- ❏ tricitrates
- ❏ tricitrates SF
- ❏ TriCor
- ❏ Tridesilon
- ❏ Tridil
- ❏ trientine
- ❏ Triesence
- ❏ trifluoperazine
- ❏ Trifluoper HCL
- ❏ trifluorothymidine
- ❏ trifluridine
- ❏ Triglide
- ❏ trihexyphenidyl
- ❏ TriHIBit
- ❏ Trikof-D
- ❏ Trilafon
- ❏ Trileptal
- ❏ Tri-Levlen
- ❏ Trilipix
- ❏ Trilisate
- ❏ Trilostane
- ❏ Tri-Luma Cream
- ❏ trimethobenzamide
- ❏ Trimethoprim
- ❏ trimetrexate
- ❏ trimipramine
- ❏ Trimox
- ❏ Trimpex
- ❏ trimipramine
- ❏ Trinalin
- ❏ TriNessa
- ❏ Tri-Nasal
- ❏ Tri-Norinyl
- ❏ Trinsicon
- ❏ Triostat
- ❏ Tripedia
- ❏ Tripelennamine
- ❏ Triphasil
- ❏ triprolidine
- ❏ Triptans
- ❏ triptorelin pamoate

## T

- ❑ Trisenox
- ❑ Trisoralen
- ❑ Tritec
- ❑ Tri-Thalmic
- ❑ Trivaris
- ❑ Trivora
- ❑ trivagizole
- ❑ Trizivir
- ❑ Trobicin
- ❑ troglitazone
- ❑ troleandomycin
- ❑ tromethamine
- ❑ Tronolane
- ❑ TrophAmine
- ❑ tropicacyl
- ❑ tropicamide
- ❑ trospium
- ❑ trospium chloride
- ❑ trovafloxacin
- ❑ Trovan
- ❑ Truphylline
- ❑ Trusopt
- ❑ Truvada
- ❑ Truxophylline
- ❑ Trypsin
- ❑ tryptophan
- ❑ Trysol
- ❑ TSPA
- ❑ T-Stat
- ❑ Tubersol
- ❑ Tucks
- ❑ Tums
- ❑ Tussafed
- ❑ Tussend
- ❑ Tussin
- ❑ Tussionex Pennkinetic
- ❑ Tussi-Organidin
- ❑ Tussizone
- ❑ TVP-1012
- ❑ Twinlab GTB Chromium
- ❑ Twinject

## T

- ❑ Twinrix
- ❑ Tygacil
- ❑ Tykerb
- ❑ Tylenol
- ❑ Tylenol caplets
- ❑ Tylenol geltabs
- ❑ Tylox
- ❑ Tyloxapol
- ❑ Tympagesic
- ❑ Typhim Vi
- ❑ tyrothrycin
- ❑ Tysabri
- ❑ Tyzeka

## U

- ❑ U-90152S
- ❑ UK-68-798
- ❑ UK 92480
- ❑ Ulcine
- ❑ Ultane
- ❑ Ultiva
- ❑ Ultrabrom
- ❑ Ultracet
- ❑ Ultra-Fiber
- ❑ Ultralente
- ❑ Ultram
- ❑ Ultrase
- ❑ Ultra-TechneKow DTE
- ❑ Ultravate
- ❑ Ultravist
- ❑ Unasyn
- ❑ undecylenic acid
- ❑ Unguentine
- ❑ Unicap
- ❑ Unicontin
- ❑ Unidor
- ❑ Unifiber
- ❑ Unipen
- ❑ Uniphyl
- ❑ Uniretic

67

| U | V |
|---|---|
| ❑ Unisom | ❑ Vaccinia |
| ❑ Unisyn | ❑ Vacuette |
| ❑ Unithroid | ❑ Vagifem |
| ❑ Uni-Tussin | ❑ Vagisil |
| ❑ Univasc | ❑ Vagistat |
| ❑ unoprostone | ❑ valacyclovir |
| ❑ Uprima | ❑ Valadol |
| ❑ urea | ❑ Valcyte |
| ❑ Ureacin | ❑ valdecoxib |
| ❑ Ureaphil | ❑ Valergen |
| ❑ Urecholine | ❑ Valerian |
| ❑ Urex | ❑ valganciclovir |
| ❑ Uricalm | ❑ Valisone |
| ❑ Uridon | ❑ Valium |
| ❑ Urimax | ❑ valproate sodium |
| ❑ Urised | ❑ valproic acid |
| ❑ Urispas | ❑ Valrelease |
| ❑ Uristat | ❑ valrubicin |
| ❑ Urobak | ❑ valsartan |
| ❑ Urobiotic 250 | ❑ Valstar |
| ❑ Urocit-K | ❑ Valtrex |
| ❑ Urodine | ❑ Vamate |
| ❑ Urodol | ❑ Vancenase |
| ❑ urofollitropin | ❑ Vanceril |
| ❑ Urogesic | ❑ Vancocin |
| ❑ Urokinase | ❑ Vancoled |
| ❑ Uro-KP-Neutral | ❑ vancomycin |
| ❑ Urolene blue | ❑ Vanex |
| ❑ Uro-Mag | ❑ Vaniqa |
| ❑ Uroplus | ❑ Vanlev |
| ❑ Uroquid-Acid | ❑ Vanos |
| ❑ Urovist Cysto | ❑ Vanoxide |
| ❑ UroXatral | ❑ Vanquish |
| ❑ Urozide | ❑ Vantas |
| ❑ Urso | ❑ Vantin |
| ❑ Urso Forte | ❑ Vaprisol |
| ❑ ursodeoxycholic acid | ❑ VAQTA |
| ❑ Ursodiol | ❑ vardenafil |
| ❑ Uvadex | ❑ varenicline |
| | ❑ Varidox |
| | ❑ Varivax |

## V

- ❑ Vascor
- ❑ Vascoray
- ❑ Vaseretic
- ❑ Vaseline
- ❑ Vaso-Lene
- ❑ Vasoplex
- ❑ Vasocidin
- ❑ VasoClear
- ❑ Vasocon
- ❑ Vasodilan
- ❑ Vasomax
- ❑ Vasopressin
- ❑ Vasovist
- ❑ Vaseretic
- ❑ Vasosulf
- ❑ Vasotec
- ❑ Vasoxyl
- ❑ Vatronol
- ❑ VCF Film
- ❑ Vectibix
- ❑ vecuronium
- ❑ Veetids
- ❑ Velban
- ❑ Velcade
- ❑ Velosulin BR
- ❑ Velsar
- ❑ Venastat
- ❑ venlafaxine
- ❑ Venofer
- ❑ Venoglobulin-S
- ❑ Ventavis
- ❑ Ventolin
- ❑ Ventolin HFA
- ❑ VePesid
- ❑ Veramyst
- ❑ Verapamil
- ❑ Verdeso
- ❑ Veregen
- ❑ Verelan
- ❑ Vermox
- ❑ Verrex

## V

- ❑ Verrusol
- ❑ Versacaps
- ❑ Versed
- ❑ Versiclear
- ❑ verteporfin
- ❑ Vertigoheel
- ❑ Vesanoid
- ❑ Vesicare
- ❑ Vexol
- ❑ VFEND
- ❑ Viactiv
- ❑ Viadur
- ❑ Viagra
- ❑ Vibramycin
- ❑ Vibra-Tabs
- ❑ Vicks
- ❑ Vicks 44D
- ❑ Vicks 44E
- ❑ Vicks Casero
- ❑ Vicks DayQuil
- ❑ Vicks Nyquil
- ❑ Vicks Sinex
- ❑ Vicks VapoRub
- ❑ Vicks VapoSteam
- ❑ Vicodin
- ❑ Vicon Forte
- ❑ Vicoprofen
- ❑ vidarabine
- ❑ Vi-Daylin ADC
- ❑ Vidaza
- ❑ Videx
- ❑ Vigabatrin
- ❑ Vigamox
- ❑ Vimpat
- ❑ vinblastine
- ❑ Vinarol
- ❑ vincristine
- ❑ vindesine
- ❑ vinorelbine
- ❑ vinpocetine
- ❑ Viokase

## V

- Vioxx
- Vira-A
- Viracept
- Viramune
- Virazole
- Viread
- Virilon
- Viroptic
- ViroSeq HIV-1
- Visicol
- Visine
- Visine-A
- Visine L.R.
- Visipaque
- Visculose
- viscum album
- Visken
- Vistaril
- Vistide
- Visudyne Photodynamic
- VISUtein
- Vitafol
- Vita-Minz
- Vitamist
- ViTelle Lurline PMS
- vitex agnus-castus
- Vitrase
- Vitrasert
- Vitravene
- Vivactil
- Viva-Drops
- Vivaglobin
- Vivarin
- Vivelle
- Vivelle-DOT
- Vivitrex
- Vivitrol
- Vivotif Berna
- VLB
- VM-26
- Volmax

## V

- Voltaren
- Vontrol
- Voriconazole
- vorinostat
- VoSol
- VP-16
- Vumon
- Vytone
- Vytorin
- Vyvanse
- VZIG

## W

- Wake-Up
- warfarin
- Wartner
- Wart-Off
- Water-Jel
- WE Allergy
- WelChol
- Wellbutrin
- Wellcovorin
- Westhroid
- Wigraine
- WinGel
- Winrgy
- WinRho SDF
- Winstrol
- Wobenzym
- Wondra
- Wycillin
- Wydase
- Wygesic
- Wymox
- Wytensin

## X

- ❏ Xalatan
- ❏ Xanax
- ❏ xanthine oxidase inhibitor
- ❏ Xcytrin
- ❏ Xeloda
- ❏ Xenaderm
- ❏ Xenadrine
- ❏ Xenazine
- ❏ Xenical
- ❏ Xerac AC
- ❏ Xero-Lube
- ❏ Xibrom
- ❏ Xience
- ❏ Xifaxan
- ❏ Xigris
- ❏ ximelagatran
- ❏ XL-3
- ❏ Xolair
- ❏ Xolegel
- ❏ Xopenex
- ❏ X-Prep
- ❏ XtremeLean
- ❏ X-Trozine
- ❏ Xylocaine
- ❏ Xylocard
- ❏ Xylometazoline
- ❏ Xyrem
- ❏ Xyntha
- ❏ Xyzal

## Y

- ❏ Yaz
- ❏ Yasmin
- ❏ YF-VAX
- ❏ Yocon
- ❏ Yodoxin
- ❏ yohimbine
- ❏ Yohimex
- ❏ Youthgenes spray
- ❏ Yutopar

## Z

- ❏ Zadaxin
- ❏ Zaditor
- ❏ zafirlukast
- ❏ Zagam
- ❏ zalcitabine
- ❏ Zaleplon
- ❏ Zanaflex
- ❏ Zanamivar
- ❏ Zanosar
- ❏ Zantac
- ❏ Zantrex
- ❏ Zantryl
- ❏ Zapex
- ❏ ZAPZYT
- ❏ Zarontin
- ❏ Zaroxolyn
- ❏ Zavesca
- ❏ Zeasorb
- ❏ zeaxanthin
- ❏ Zebeta
- ❏ Zebrax
- ❏ Zebutal
- ❏ Zeel
- ❏ Zefazone
- ❏ Zegerid
- ❏ Zelapar
- ❏ Zelnorm
- ❏ Zemaira
- ❏ Zemplar
- ❏ Zemuron
- ❏ Zenapax
- ❏ ZenChent
- ❏ Zephrex
- ❏ Zerit
- ❏ Zeroxin
- ❏ Zestoretic
- ❏ Zestril
- ❏ Zetar
- ❏ Zetia
- ❏ Zetran
- ❏ Zevalin

## Z

- ❑ Ziac
- ❑ Ziagen
- ❑ Ziana
- ❑ Zicam
- ❑ zidovudine
- ❑ Zilactin
- ❑ zileuton
- ❑ Zinacef
- ❑ zinc
- ❑ zinc bisglycinate
- ❑ zinc oxide
- ❑ zinc pyrithione
- ❑ zinc sulfate
- ❑ Zincfrin
- ❑ Zinecard
- ❑ Zingo
- ❑ ziprasidone mesylate
- ❑ Zithromax
- ❑ Zmax
- ❑ Zocor
- ❑ Zofran
- ❑ Zoladex
- ❑ zoledronate
- ❑ zoledronic acid
- ❑ Zolinza
- ❑ Zometa
- ❑ Zolmitriptan
- ❑ Zoloft
- ❑ zolpidem tartrate
- ❑ Zolpimist
- ❑ Zolyse
- ❑ Zometa
- ❑ Zomig
- ❑ Zomig-ZMT
- ❑ Zonalon
- ❑ Zonegran
- ❑ zonisamide
- ❑ Zorbtive
- ❑ Zorprin
- ❑ Zostavax
- ❑ Zosyn

## Z

- ❑ Zotarolimus
- ❑ Zoto-HC eardrops
- ❑ Zotrim
- ❑ Zotrix
- ❑ Zovia
- ❑ Zovirax
- ❑ Zyban
- ❑ Zydone
- ❑ Zyflo
- ❑ Zyflo CR
- ❑ Zylet
- ❑ Zyloprim
- ❑ Zymar
- ❑ Zymase
- ❑ Zymenol
- ❑ Zyprexa
- ❑ Zyrtec
- ❑ Zyrtec-D
- ❑ Zyvox

| ■ | A | | ■ | A |

■ **AIDS**

- ❑ abacavir
- ❑ Agenerase
- ❑ AGT 088
- ❑ Aidsvax
- ❑ alitretinoin
- ❑ AmBisome
- ❑ AMD-070
- ❑ Amdoxovir
- ❑ Ampligen
- ❑ amprenavir
- ❑ Ao-Zidovudine
- ❑ Aptivus
- ❑ Aralen
- ❑ atazanavir
- ❑ atovaquone
- ❑ Atripla
- ❑ AVX101
- ❑ AZT
- ❑ azidothymidine
- ❑ Bactrim
- ❑ Biaxin
- ❑ Biozole
- ❑ CCR5 blockade
- ❑ CCR5 inhibitors
- ❑ cidofovir
- ❑ Combivir
- ❑ co-trimoxazole
- ❑ Crixivan
- ❑ cyanocobalamin
- ❑ Cytovene
- ❑ d4t
- ❑ DAPD
- ❑ Dapsone
- ❑ Daraprim
- ❑ darunavir
- ❑ daunorubicin
- ❑ DaunoXome
- ❑ ddC
- ❑ delavirdine
- ❑ didanosine

- ❑ Diflucan
- ❑ Doxil
- ❑ Drabinol
- ❑ efavirenz
- ❑ emtricitabine
- ❑ Emtriva
- ❑ ENF (T-20)
- ❑ Enfuvirtide
- ❑ Epivir
- ❑ Epzicom
- ❑ ethionamide
- ❑ etravirine
- ❑ EZ MedTest
- ❑ Famvir
- ❑ Flumadine
- ❑ Formivirsen
- ❑ Fortovase
- ❑ Fosamprenavir
- ❑ foscarnete
- ❑ Foscavir
- ❑ fusion inhibitors
- ❑ Fuzeon
- ❑ ganciclovir
- ❑ HPA-23
- ❑ Hivid
- ❑ indinavir
- ❑ Infergen
- ❑ Integrase inhibitors
- ❑ Intelence
- ❑ Interferon Alfa-N3
- ❑ Intron A
- ❑ Invirase
- ❑ Isentress
- ❑ Kaletra
- ❑ lamivudine
- ❑ Lexiva
- ❑ lopinavir
- ❑ maraviroc
- ❑ Marinol
- ❑ Megace
- ❑ megestrol

73

## A

- ❑ Mepron
- ❑ methylprednisolone
- ❑ Mycobutin
- ❑ Nascobal
- ❑ NebuPen
- ❑ nelfinavir
- ❑ Neutrexin
- ❑ NFV
- ❑ Norvir
- ❑ Novo-AZT
- ❑ Noxafil
- ❑ Octagam
- ❑ Panretin
- ❑ Paser
- ❑ Pentacarinat
- ❑ Pentam
- ❑ pentamidine
- ❑ Peptidic PI
- ❑ Pneumopent
- ❑ Pneumovax
- ❑ Pnu-Imune
- ❑ Podofilox
- ❑ podophyllin
- ❑ posaconazole
- ❑ Prezista
- ❑ Priftin
- ❑ Racivir
- ❑ raltegravir
- ❑ Rebetron
- ❑ Reiki
- ❑ Remune
- ❑ Rescriptor
- ❑ Retrovir
- ❑ Reyataz
- ❑ Rifadin
- ❑ Rifamate
- ❑ Rifater
- ❑ ritonavir
- ❑ RO-033-4649
- ❑ Roferon A
- ❑ saquinavir

## A

- ❑ Sculptra
- ❑ Selzentry
- ❑ Septra
- ❑ shikonin
- ❑ Sporanox
- ❑ stavudine
- ❑ Streptomycin sulfate
- ❑ Sustiva
- ❑ Symmetrel
- ❑ Synagis
- ❑ T-1249
- ❑ tenofovir disoproxil fumarate
- ❑ tipranavir
- ❑ TMC-114
- ❑ TNX-355
- ❑ Trecator-SC
- ❑ trimetrexate
- ❑ Trizivir
- ❑ Truvada
- ❑ Valcyte
- ❑ valganciclovir
- ❑ Valtrex
- ❑ Videx
- ❑ Viracept
- ❑ Viramune
- ❑ Viread
- ❑ ViroSeq HIV-1
- ❑ Vistide
- ❑ Vitrasert
- ❑ Vitravene
- ❑ Yodoxin
- ❑ zalcitabine
- ❑ Zerit
- ❑ Ziagen
- ❑ zidovudine
- ❑ Zithromax
- ❑ Zovirax

## ■ ALZHEIMER'S DISEASE

- ❑ ampakine
- ❑ Aricept

| ■ | A |
|---|---|

- ❑ atomoxetine
- ❑ Cognex
- ❑ Concerta
- ❑ CX-516
- ❑ dexmethylphenidate
- ❑ donepezil
- ❑ Exelon
- ❑ Focalin
- ❑ galantamine Hbr
- ❑ MEM 1414
- ❑ memantine
- ❑ Metadate
- ❑ Methylin
- ❑ methylphenidate
- ❑ Namenda
- ❑ Phenserine
- ❑ Razadyne
- ❑ Reminyl
- ❑ Riphenidate
- ❑ Ritalin
- ❑ rivastigmine
- ❑ SGS742
- ❑ Strattera
- ❑ Tacrine
- ❑ Trizivir

## ■ ANALGESICS

- ❑ Abreva
- ❑ Acephen
- ❑ Aceta
- ❑ acetaminophen
- ❑ acrivastine
- ❑ Actamin
- ❑ Actiq
- ❑ Acubead
- ❑ Adnexsia
- ❑ Advil
- ❑ Advil Liqui-Gels
- ❑ Aflaxin
- ❑ Aggrenox
- ❑ Aleve

| ■ | A |
|---|---|

- ❑ Alfenta
- ❑ alfentanil
- ❑ Alka-Seltzer
- ❑ Allay
- ❑ almotriptan malate
- ❑ Alumadrine
- ❑ Amerge
- ❑ Aminofem
- ❑ Anabar
- ❑ Anacin
- ❑ Anakinra
- ❑ Anaprox
- ❑ Anbesol
- ❑ Aniledrine
- ❑ Anexsia
- ❑ Anolor
- ❑ Apacet
- ❑ Apamide
- ❑ APAP/Codeine
- ❑ APC
- ❑ Atasol
- ❑ Arth DR
- ❑ Arthrotec
- ❑ Arth-Rx
- ❑ Arthur Itis
- ❑ Ascriptin
- ❑ Aspercreme
- ❑ Aspergum
- ❑ aspirin
- ❑ Astramorph
- ❑ Atretol
- ❑ Auroto Otic
- ❑ Avinza
- ❑ Axert
- ❑ Axotal
- ❑ Azdone
- ❑ Backaid
- ❑ Bactine
- ❑ Bancap
- ❑ Banesin
- ❑ Bayer

| ■ A | ■ A |
|---|---|
| ❑ Benadryl | ❑ Damason |
| ❑ Benadryl-D | ❑ Dapa |
| ❑ BeneJoint | ❑ Darvocet-A 500 |
| ❑ Bengay | ❑ Darvocet-N |
| ❑ benzocaine | ❑ Darvon |
| ❑ Bextra | ❑ Datril |
| ❑ Bicozene | ❑ Daypro |
| ❑ Bluboro | ❑ Demerol |
| ❑ Bufferin | ❑ DepoDur |
| ❑ Buffets | ❑ DepoFoam |
| ❑ Bupap | ❑ Depomorphine |
| ❑ Buprenex | ❑ dezocine |
| ❑ buprenorphine | ❑ diclofenac |
| ❑ butalbital | ❑ diflunisal |
| ❑ butorphanol | ❑ difluprednate |
| ❑ Campo-Phenique | ❑ Dilaudid |
| ❑ capsaicin cream | ❑ Disalcid |
| ❑ carispoprodol | ❑ Doan's |
| ❑ Carmex | ❑ Dolobid |
| ❑ Cataflam | ❑ Dolacet |
| ❑ Celebrex | ❑ Dolagesic |
| ❑ Cepacol | ❑ Dolene-AP |
| ❑ Capzasin-P | ❑ Dolorac |
| ❑ carbamazepine | ❑ Dristan |
| ❑ Carbatrol | ❑ Drocade/Aspirin |
| ❑ Cetacaine | ❑ Doublecap |
| ❑ Chloraseptic | ❑ Duraclon |
| ❑ chlorzoxazone | ❑ Duract |
| ❑ Clinoril | ❑ Duragesic |
| ❑ clonidine | ❑ Duramorph |
| ❑ Codamine | ❑ Durezol |
| ❑ codeine | ❑ Easprin |
| ❑ Codrex | ❑ EC-Naprosyn |
| ❑ Co-Gesic | ❑ Ecotrin |
| ❑ Combunox | ❑ E-Lor |
| ❑ Compoz | ❑ Emcodeine |
| ❑ Comtrex | ❑ Empirin |
| ❑ Congespirin | ❑ Empracet |
| ❑ Coricidin | ❑ Emtec |
| ❑ Cox-2 inhibitor | ❑ Enbrel |
| ❑ Dalgan | ❑ Endocet |

| | A | | | A |
|---|---|---|---|---|

- ❑ enteric aspirin
- ❑ Equagesic
- ❑ ESGIC
- ❑ etanercept
- ❑ ethyl aminobenzoate
- ❑ etodolac
- ❑ etodolic acid
- ❑ Excedrin
- ❑ Excedrin Quicktabs
- ❑ Exdol
- ❑ Extendryl
- ❑ EZ III
- ❑ Ezol
- ❑ Feldene
- ❑ felodipine
- ❑ Femcet
- ❑ fentanyl
- ❑ fentanyl citrate
- ❑ Fentora
- ❑ Feridex I.V.
- ❑ ferrous fumarate
- ❑ ferrous gluconate
- ❑ ferrous sulfate
- ❑ ferumoxides
- ❑ Feverall
- ❑ fexofenadine
- ❑ Fiberall
- ❑ Fiber-Lax
- ❑ filgrastim
- ❑ Finasteride
- ❑ Floricet
- ❑ Fiorinal
- ❑ Fiortal
- ❑ Flagyl
- ❑ Flatulex
- ❑ flavoxate
- ❑ flecainide
- ❑ Flector
- ❑ Fleet Babylax
- ❑ Fleet Bisacodyl
- ❑ Fleet Enema

- ❑ Fleet Phospho Soda
- ❑ Flexall
- ❑ Flexaphen
- ❑ Flo-Coat
- ❑ floctafenine
- ❑ Flolan
- ❑ Flomax
- ❑ Flonase
- ❑ Florone
- ❑ Flovent
- ❑ Floxan
- ❑ floxuridine
- ❑ Flubiprofen
- ❑ fluconazole
- ❑ flucytosine
- ❑ fludarabine
- ❑ fludrocortisone
- ❑ flumazenil
- ❑ flunisolide
- ❑ fluocinolone
- ❑ fluocinonide
- ❑ Fluogen
- ❑ Fluonid
- ❑ Fluoracaine
- ❑ fluorescein
- ❑ fluoride
- ❑ fluorometholone
- ❑ fluorouracil
- ❑ Fluothane
- ❑ fluoxetine
- ❑ fluoxymesterone
- ❑ fluphenazine
- ❑ flurandrenolide
- ❑ flurazepam
- ❑ flurbiprofen
- ❑ Fluress
- ❑ flutamide
- ❑ fluticasone & salmeterol
- ❑ fluvastatin
- ❑ fluvoxamine
- ❑ Fluzone

| ☐ A | ☐ A |
|---|---|
| ☐ Frova | ☐ lidocaine |
| ☐ frovatriptan | ☐ Lidoderm patch |
| ☐ FUDR | ☐ Liquiprin |
| ☐ gaba analog | ☐ Lodine |
| ☐ Gelprin | ☐ Lorcet |
| ☐ Genapap | ☐ Lortab |
| ☐ glycyrrhetinic acid | ☐ Lurline |
| ☐ Goody's | ☐ Lyrica |
| ☐ Halfprin | ☐ Margesic |
| ☐ Healthprin | ☐ Maxalt-MLT |
| ☐ Heet liniment | ☐ Maxidone |
| ☐ Herpecin-L | ☐ Medigesic |
| ☐ Hyalgan | ☐ mefenamic acid |
| ☐ Hycet | ☐ meprobamate |
| ☐ Hycomed | ☐ Mepergan |
| ☐ Hycomine | ☐ Meperidine |
| ☐ Hycopap | ☐ Methadone |
| ☐ Hydrocet | ☐ Medastron |
| ☐ hydrocodone bitartrate | ☐ Midol |
| ☐ hydrocodone polistirex | ☐ Midrin |
| ☐ Hydrogesic | ☐ MigraHealth |
| ☐ hydromorphone | ☐ Migra spray |
| ☐ HY-PHEN | ☐ milnacipran |
| ☐ ibuprofen | ☐ Mobigesic |
| ☐ Indocin | ☐ Mono-Gesic |
| ☐ Infumorph | ☐ morphine sulfate |
| ☐ Ionsys transdermal | ☐ Motrin |
| ☐ Kadian | ☐ MS Contin |
| ☐ Kank-A | ☐ MSIR |
| ☐ ketoprolac | ☐ MT100 |
| ☐ Kineret | ☐ Myoflex |
| ☐ Kneerelief | ☐ nalbuphine |
| ☐ L.M.X.4 cream | ☐ Nalfon |
| ☐ L.M.X.5 cream | ☐ naloxone |
| ☐ Lanotec/Codeine | ☐ Naprelan |
| ☐ Laudanum | ☐ Naprosyn |
| ☐ Legatrin | ☐ naratriptan |
| ☐ Levo-Dromoran | ☐ Neopap |
| ☐ Levoprome | ☐ nepafenac |
| ☐ levophanol | ☐ Neurontin |
| ☐ Lexidronam | ☐ Nevanac |

| ■ A | ■ A |
|---|---|
| ❑ Norco | ❑ pentazocine |
| ❑ Norel | ❑ Percocet |
| ❑ Norflex | ❑ Percodan |
| ❑ Norgesic | ❑ Percogesic |
| ❑ Novitra | ❑ Percolone |
| ❑ Novo-AC | ❑ Perform |
| ❑ Novogesic | ❑ Phenaphen/Codeine |
| ❑ Nubain | ❑ Phenergan |
| ❑ Nucofed | ❑ phenol |
| ❑ Numorphan | ❑ Phrenilin Forte |
| ❑ Nupercainal | ❑ Polygesic |
| ❑ Onset | ❑ Ponstel |
| ❑ Opana | ❑ Pregabalin |
| ❑ Orabase | ❑ Premsyn |
| ❑ Orajel | ❑ Prialt |
| ❑ Oramorph | ❑ Prid |
| ❑ Oraphen | ❑ Prodium |
| ❑ OraVescent Fentanyl | ❑ Propacet |
| ❑ Orlamm | ❑ Pro Pox/APAP |
| ❑ Ornex | ❑ propoxyphene |
| ❑ orphenadrine | ❑ propoxyphene napsylate |
| ❑ orphengesic | ❑ Protid |
| ❑ Orudis | ❑ Pyregesic |
| ❑ Oruvail | ❑ Pyridium |
| ❑ Oxycet | ❑ Quadramet |
| ❑ Oxycodan | ❑ Ralivia |
| ❑ oxycodone | ❑ Redutemp |
| ❑ OxyContin | ❑ Relafen |
| ❑ Oxy-Fast | ❑ Releev |
| ❑ Oxy-IR | ❑ Repan |
| ❑ oxymorphone | ❑ Relpax |
| ❑ Pacaps | ❑ Rid-A-Pain |
| ❑ Palladone | ❑ Robaxin |
| ❑ Pamprin | ❑ rofecoxib |
| ❑ Panacet | ❑ Roxanol |
| ❑ Panadol | ❑ Roxicet |
| ❑ Panasal | ❑ Roxicodone |
| ❑ Panlor | ❑ Roxiflex |
| ❑ Paraflex | ❑ Roxilox |
| ❑ Parafon Forte | ❑ Roxiprin |
| ❑ PC Cap | ❑ Ryzolt |

## A

- Saleto
- Salflex
- Salonpas
- Sansert
- Sativex
- Sedapap
- Semprex
- Sinarest
- Sine-Aid
- Sinulin
- Sinutab
- Snaplets
- Soma Compound
- Stadol
- Stagesic
- Stanback
- St. Joseph Aspirin
- Sublimaze
- Sudafed
- Sufenta
- sufentanil
- sumatriptan
- Sunril
- Supac
- Suppap
- Synalgos
- Synvisc
- Talacen
- Talwin
- Tanac
- Tapanol
- Tapentadol
- Tegretol
- Tempra
- Tencon
- Theragesic
- ThermaCare
- Tolectin
- Topricin
- Toradol
- Tramadol

## A

- Tranadik
- Traumeel
- Trexima
- Treximet
- Trilisate
- Tylaprin/Codeine
- Tylenol
- Tylenol caplets
- Tylenol geltabs
- Tylox
- Ugesic
- Ultiva
- Ultracet
- Ultragesic
- Ulram
- valdecoxib
- Valorin
- Vanacet
- Vanquish
- Vapocet
- Veganin
- Vendone
- Vicodin
- Vicoprofen
- Vioxx
- ViTelle Lurline PMS
- Voltaren
- Wygesic
- Zebutal
- Zeel
- Zilactin
- Zingo
- Zostrix
- Zydone

### ■ ANESTHETICS
- Akten
- Americaine
- Amidate
- Amytal
- Anectine

| ■ | A | | ■ | A |
|---|---|---|---|---|

- ❑ Anestacon
- ❑ Aquachloral
- ❑ Aquavan
- ❑ Aramine
- ❑ Articaine
- ❑ Astracaine
- ❑ atracurium
- ❑ Avertin
- ❑ Bactine
- ❑ benzocaine
- ❑ Benzodent
- ❑ Blockain
- ❑ brevital, sodium
- ❑ Brietal
- ❑ bupivacaine
- ❑ Butadiene
- ❑ Carbocaine
- ❑ Cetacaine
- ❑ Chirocaine
- ❑ chloral hydrate
- ❑ chloroethane
- ❑ chloroform
- ❑ chloroprocaine
- ❑ cisatracurium besylate
- ❑ Citanest
- ❑ curare
- ❑ Cyclaine
- ❑ cyclohexane
- ❑ cyclopentane
- ❑ cyclopropane
- ❑ Dalcaine
- ❑ Dentapaine
- ❑ Dent-Zel-Ite
- ❑ desflurane
- ❑ diethyl ether
- ❑ Diprivan
- ❑ divinyl oxide
- ❑ doxacurium
- ❑ doxapram
- ❑ Droperidol
- ❑ Duranest

- ❑ Dyclone
- ❑ dyclonine
- ❑ EMLA
- ❑ enflurane
- ❑ ether
- ❑ Ethocaine
- ❑ Ethrane
- ❑ ethyl aminobenzoate
- ❑ ethyl ether
- ❑ Ethylene
- ❑ etidocaine
- ❑ Fentanyl
- ❑ Fleet Anorectal
- ❑ flumazenil
- ❑ flunitrazepam
- ❑ Fluothane
- ❑ Fluro-Ethyl
- ❑ Forane
- ❑ fospropofol
- ❑ Halothane
- ❑ Hemorid
- ❑ Hexylcaine
- ❑ Hurricaine
- ❑ Innovar
- ❑ Ketalar
- ❑ Inapsine
- ❑ Iontophoretic
- ❑ Isocaine
- ❑ isoflurane
- ❑ L-Caine
- ❑ Lanacane
- ❑ levobupivacaine
- ❑ lidocaine
- ❑ Lidoject
- ❑ LidoSite
- ❑ Lusedra
- ❑ Marcaine
- ❑ Mepergan
- ❑ meperidine
- ❑ mepivacaine
- ❑ metaraminol

| | A |
|---|---|

- methohexital
- methoxamine
- midazolam
- Mivacron
- mivacurium
- Naropin
- Nesacaine
- Nimbex
- Noctec
- Norcuron
- Novocain
- novochlorhydrate
- Numzident
- Num-Zit-Gel
- Nupercainal
- Nuromax
- Octocaine
- On-Q
- Ophthaine
- Oraqix
- OraVerse
- pancuronium
- Pavulon
- Penthrane
- Polocaine
- Pontocaine
- Preject
- Preparation H
- prilocaine
- procaine
- ProctoFoam
- propofo
- Raplon
- remifentanil
- Robinul
- rocuronium
- Rohypnol
- Romazicon
- ropivacaine
- Sarapin
- S-Caine Peel

| | A |
|---|---|

- Sensorcaine
- Sevoflurane
- sodium brevital
- sodium pentothal
- Sojourn Sevoflurane
- Solarcaine
- Sublimaze
- succinylcholine
- Suprane
- surital sodium
- Synera
- tetracaine
- thiopental sodium
- Tracrium
- Tronolane
- Tucks
- Ultane
- Ultiva
- Ultracaine
- Vasoxyl
- vecuronium
- Versed
- Xylocaine
- Zemuron
- Zilactin

## ■ ANTACIDS

- AcipHex
- Alka-Seltzer
- Alternagel
- aluminum hydroxide
- aluminum magnesia
- Amitone
- Amphojel
- Axid
- Beano
- bethanechol
- Bisodol
- Brioschi Powder
- calcium carbonate
- Camalox

| ■ A |
| --- |

- ❑ Carbamine
- ❑ Carafate
- ❑ cimetidine
- ❑ Ceo Two
- ❑ Chooz
- ❑ citrocarbonate
- ❑ Dicarbosil
- ❑ Di-Gel
- ❑ esomeprazole
- ❑ Famodine
- ❑ famotidine
- ❑ Fluxid
- ❑ GasAid
- ❑ Gas-X
- ❑ Gaviscon
- ❑ Gelcid
- ❑ Gelusil
- ❑ H2 Blockers
- ❑ Kolantyl
- ❑ Kudrox
- ❑ lansoprazole
- ❑ Little Tummys
- ❑ Maalox
- ❑ Mag-al
- ❑ Magnatril
- ❑ magnesium carbonate
- ❑ magnesium hydroxide
- ❑ magnesium oxide
- ❑ magnesium trisilicate
- ❑ metoclopramide
- ❑ Milk of Magnesia
- ❑ Mylanta
- ❑ Mylicon
- ❑ Nephrox
- ❑ Neutrolox
- ❑ Nexium
- ❑ Nulev
- ❑ omeprazole
- ❑ Oxaine
- ❑ pantoprazole
- ❑ Pepcid

| ■ A |
| --- |

- ❑ Pepcid AC
- ❑ Pepto-Bismol
- ❑ Phillips Milk of Magnesia
- ❑ Prilosec
- ❑ Prilosec OTC
- ❑ prokinetics
- ❑ Protonix
- ❑ proton pump inhibitors
- ❑ rabeprazole
- ❑ ranitidine
- ❑ Rapinex
- ❑ Reglan
- ❑ Riopan
- ❑ Rolaids
- ❑ Rolaids softchews
- ❑ sucralftate
- ❑ Tagamet
- ❑ Tegaserod
- ❑ Titralac
- ❑ Tums
- ❑ urecholine
- ❑ Zantac
- ❑ Zegerid
- ❑ Zelnorm

**■ ANTIBIOTICS**

- ❑ Achromycin
- ❑ Adoxa
- ❑ Advicor
- ❑ Amikacin
- ❑ Amikin
- ❑ Ancef
- ❑ Ancobon
- ❑ Alpha-Proteinase
- ❑ anidulafungin
- ❑ Ansamycin
- ❑ Antibiopto
- ❑ Aralast NP
- ❑ Arcalyst
- ❑ atovaquone
- ❑ Atrosept

| ■ | A |
| --- | --- |

| ■ | A |
| --- | --- |

- ❑ Augmentin
- ❑ Aureomycin
- ❑ Avelox
- ❑ Azactam
- ❑ AzaSite
- ❑ aztreonam
- ❑ azafluoroquinolone
- ❑ azithromycin
- ❑ Aztreonam
- ❑ bacampicillin
- ❑ Bacitracin
- ❑ Bactine
- ❑ Bactrim
- ❑ beta-lactame
- ❑ Biaxin
- ❑ Bicillin
- ❑ Biocef
- ❑ Bio-Triple
- ❑ biskalcitrate
- ❑ Blenoxane
- ❑ bleomycin
- ❑ Bleph-10
- ❑ Cancidas
- ❑ Capastat
- ❑ capreomycin
- ❑ carbenicillin indanyl
- ❑ caspofungin
- ❑ Ceclor
- ❑ Cedax
- ❑ cefaclor
- ❑ Cefadyl
- ❑ cefadroxil
- ❑ cefamandole naftate
- ❑ cefazolin
- ❑ cefdinir
- ❑ cefditoren
- ❑ cefepime
- ❑ cefixime
- ❑ Cefotan
- ❑ cefotaxime
- ❑ cefotetan disodium

- ❑ cefoxitin
- ❑ cefpodoxime
- ❑ cefprozil
- ❑ ceftazidime
- ❑ ceftibuten
- ❑ Ceftin
- ❑ ceftizoxime
- ❑ ceftriaxone
- ❑ cefuroxime
- ❑ cefzil
- ❑ cephradine
- ❑ cephalexin
- ❑ cephalosporin
- ❑ Cephalothin
- ❑ Cephapirin
- ❑ Cephradine
- ❑ Ceptaz
- ❑ Cerubidine
- ❑ Chibroxin
- ❑ chloramphenicol
- ❑ Chloromycetin
- ❑ Chlorocol
- ❑ Chlorofair
- ❑ Chloroptic
- ❑ Cidomycin
- ❑ Ciloxan
- ❑ Cinobac
- ❑ cinoxacin
- ❑ Cipro
- ❑ ciprofloxacin
- ❑ Claforan
- ❑ clarithromycin
- ❑ Cleocin
- ❑ Clindagel
- ❑ Cloxacillin
- ❑ Cloxapen
- ❑ colistimethate
- ❑ Colistin
- ❑ Coly-Mycin
- ❑ Cosmegen
- ❑ dactinomycin

| ■ A | ■ A |
|---|---|
| ❑ Daflopristin | ❑ flucytosine |
| ❑ Daraprim | ❑ fluoroquinolone |
| ❑ DaunoXome | ❑ fomivirsen |
| ❑ Declomycin | ❑ fosfomycin |
| ❑ demeclocycline | ❑ Fortaz |
| ❑ dicloxacillin | ❑ Fulvicin |
| ❑ Diflucan | ❑ Furadantin |
| ❑ dirithromycin | ❑ Furalan |
| ❑ DisperMox | ❑ Furan |
| ❑ Dolsed | ❑ Furanite |
| ❑ Doribax | ❑ furazolidone |
| ❑ doripenem | ❑ Furoxone |
| ❑ Doryx | ❑ fusidic acid |
| ❑ Doxil | ❑ Gantrisin |
| ❑ Doxorubicin | ❑ Garamycin |
| ❑ doxycycline calcium | ❑ Gatifloxacin |
| ❑ doxycycline hyclate | ❑ gemifloxacin mesylate |
| ❑ doxycycline monohydrate | ❑ Genoptic |
| ❑ Dual | ❑ Gentacidin |
| ❑ Duricef | ❑ Gentafair |
| ❑ Dycill | ❑ Gentak |
| ❑ Dynabac | ❑ gentamycin |
| ❑ Dynacin | ❑ Gentrasul |
| ❑ Dynapen | ❑ Geocillin |
| ❑ Econochlor | ❑ Geopen |
| ❑ E-Mycin | ❑ G-Myticin |
| ❑ enoxacin | ❑ Gramicidin |
| ❑ E.E.S. | ❑ grepafloxacin |
| ❑ ertapenem | ❑ Grisactin |
| ❑ Eryc | ❑ griseofulvin |
| ❑ Ery-Ped | ❑ Gris-PEG |
| ❑ Ery-Tab | ❑ Gyne-Sulf |
| ❑ Erythrocin | ❑ Helizide |
| ❑ erythromycin ethylsuccinate | ❑ Herpetrol |
| ❑ Eryzole | ❑ Hiprex |
| ❑ Factive | ❑ Idamycin |
| ❑ Femguard | ❑ Ilosone |
| ❑ Fenicol | ❑ Ilotycin |
| ❑ Flagyl | ❑ imipenem |
| ❑ Floxin | ❑ Invanz |
| ❑ fluconazole | ❑ Iquix |

| ■ A | ■ A |
|---|---|
| ❑ Jenamicin | ❑ Mithracin |
| ❑ Kanamycin | ❑ Mitomycin |
| ❑ Kantrex | ❑ Monocid |
| ❑ Keflex | ❑ Monodox |
| ❑ Keftab | ❑ Monurol |
| ❑ Kefurox | ❑ Moxatag |
| ❑ Kefzol | ❑ moxifloxacin |
| ❑ Kenalog | ❑ Mutamycin |
| ❑ Ketek | ❑ Mycamine |
| ❑ ketoconazole | ❑ Mycobutin |
| ❑ Lamisil | ❑ Mycolog |
| ❑ lansoprazole | ❑ Nafcillin |
| ❑ Levaquin | ❑ nalidixic acid |
| ❑ Levofloxacin | ❑ Nebcin |
| ❑ Lincocin | ❑ NegGram |
| ❑ linezolid | ❑ Neocidin |
| ❑ linosamides | ❑ NeoDecadron |
| ❑ lomefloxacin | ❑ neomycin |
| ❑ Lorabid | ❑ Neosporin |
| ❑ loracarbef | ❑ Neotal |
| ❑ Loridine | ❑ Neotricin |
| ❑ Lyphocin | ❑ Netromycin |
| ❑ Macrobid | ❑ Neutrexin |
| ❑ macrolides | ❑ Nipent |
| ❑ Macrodantin | ❑ nitrofurantoin |
| ❑ mandelamine | ❑ norfloxacin |
| ❑ Mandol | ❑ Noroxin |
| ❑ Maximime | ❑ Novantrone |
| ❑ Maxaquin | ❑ Noxafil |
| ❑ Mefoxin | ❑ Nystatin |
| ❑ Menactra | ❑ Ocu-Chlor |
| ❑ Mepron | ❑ Ocuflox |
| ❑ meropenem | ❑ Ocu-Mycin |
| ❑ Merrem | ❑ Ocu-Spor |
| ❑ methenamine | ❑ Ocu-Sulf |
| ❑ metronidazole | ❑ Ocutricin |
| ❑ Mezlin | ❑ ofloxacin |
| ❑ mezlocillin | ❑ oleandomycin |
| ❑ micafungin | ❑ Omnicef |
| ❑ Minocin | ❑ Omnipen |
| ❑ minocycline | ❑ Ophthacet |

| ■ A | ■ A |
|---|---|
| ❑ Oxacillin | ❑ Rubex |
| ❑ oxytetracycline | ❑ Septra |
| ❑ oxacillin | ❑ Seromycin |
| ❑ Pathocil | ❑ sodium sulamyd |
| ❑ PCE | ❑ Sopramycetin |
| ❑ Pediazole | ❑ sparfloxacin |
| ❑ Penetrex | ❑ spectinomycin |
| ❑ penicillin | ❑ Spectracef |
| ❑ Pentamycetin | ❑ Spectrobid |
| ❑ Pen-Vee | ❑ Spectro-Chlor |
| ❑ peptides | ❑ Spectro-Genta |
| ❑ peptolides | ❑ Spectro-Sporin |
| ❑ Permapen | ❑ Spectro-Sulf |
| ❑ Pfizerpen | ❑ spiramycin |
| ❑ phosphomycin | ❑ Sporanox |
| ❑ piperacillin | ❑ Staticin |
| ❑ Pipracil | ❑ Streptomycin |
| ❑ Plexion | ❑ Sulf 10 |
| ❑ P.N. Ophthalmic | ❑ sulfacetamide |
| ❑ polymyxin | ❑ sulfacytine |
| ❑ polypeptide | ❑ sulfadiazine |
| ❑ Polysporin | ❑ Sulfair |
| ❑ Polytrim | ❑ sulfabenzamide |
| ❑ posaconazole | ❑ Sulfa-Gyn |
| ❑ Prevpac | ❑ sulfamethoprim |
| ❑ Primaxin | ❑ sulfamethoxazole |
| ❑ Primsol | ❑ Sulfatrim |
| ❑ Proloprim | ❑ Sulfa-Trip |
| ❑ Pylera | ❑ Sulfamide |
| ❑ quinolone | ❑ Sulfex |
| ❑ Raxar | ❑ sulfisoxazole |
| ❑ Regasporin | ❑ sulfonamide |
| ❑ rifabutin | ❑ Sumycin |
| ❑ Rifadin | ❑ Suprax |
| ❑ Rifamate | ❑ Synercid |
| ❑ rifampin | ❑ TAO |
| ❑ Rifatar | ❑ Tazicef |
| ❑ rifaximin | ❑ Tazidime |
| ❑ rilonacept | ❑ telithromycin |
| ❑ Rocephin | ❑ Tequin |
| ❑ Rovamycine | ❑ Terra-Cortril |

| ■ A | ■ A |
|---|---|
| ❑ Terramycin | ❑ Xifaxan |
| ❑ tetracycline | ❑ Xigris |
| ❑ Ticar | ❑ Zartan |
| ❑ ticarcillin | ❑ Veetids |
| ❑ Tifacogin | ❑ Zefazone |
| ❑ Timentin | ❑ Zinacef |
| ❑ Tindamax | ❑ Zolicef |
| ❑ tinidazole | ❑ Zefazone |
| ❑ TOBI | ❑ Zinacerf |
| ❑ TobraDex | ❑ Zithromax |
| ❑ Tobramycin | ❑ Zmax |
| ❑ triamcinolone | ❑ Zosyn |
| ❑ Tribiotic | ❑ Zotrim |
| ❑ trimethoprim | ❑ Zygam |
| ❑ Trimpex | ❑ Zyvox |
| ❑ Tri-Ophthalmic | |
| ❑ Tri-Thalmic | |
| ❑ troleandomycin | **■ANTI-COAGULANTS** |
| ❑ Trovan | ❑ Abbokinase |
| ❑ T-Stat | ❑ Abbokinase Open-Cath |
| ❑ Trysul | ❑ acetylsalicylic acid |
| ❑ Unasyn | ❑ Acenocoumarol |
| ❑ Urex | ❑ alteplase |
| ❑ Uricalm | ❑ Ancrod |
| ❑ Urised | ❑ Angiomax |
| ❑ Urobiotic | ❑ Anisindione |
| ❑ Uroplus | ❑ argatroban |
| ❑ Uroquid | ❑ Arixtra |
| ❑ Valstar | ❑ Ascriptin |
| ❑ Vancocin | ❑ aspirin |
| ❑ Vancoled | ❑ bivalirudin |
| ❑ vancomycin | ❑ Bufferin |
| ❑ Vantin | ❑ calciparine |
| ❑ Vectrin | ❑ Cathflo Activase |
| ❑ Veetids | ❑ Coumadin |
| ❑ Velosef | ❑ dalteparin |
| ❑ Vibramycin | ❑ danaparoid |
| ❑ Vigtravene | ❑ Dicumarol |
| ❑ Viroptic | ❑ dipyridamole |
| ❑ Wycillin | ❑ enoxaparin |
| ❑ Wymox | ❑ enteric aspirin |

| ■ | A |
|---|---|

- ☐ Exanta
- ☐ fondaparinux
- ☐ Fragmin
- ☐ Heparin
- ☐ Kabikinase
- ☐ Lepirudin
- ☐ Liquaemin
- ☐ Lovenox
- ☐ Miradon
- ☐ Normiflo
- ☐ Orgaran
- ☐ Persantine
- ☐ Refludan
- ☐ Sintrom
- ☐ TPA
- ☐ Urokinase
- ☐ warfarin
- ☐ ximelagatran

## ■ ANTIDOTES

- ☐ acamprosate
- ☐ Acetadote
- ☐ acetylcysteine
- ☐ Actidose
- ☐ Actidose-Aqua
- ☐ activated charcoal
- ☐ amyl nitrate
- ☐ Antabuse
- ☐ Antilirium
- ☐ Antizol
- ☐ ATNNA
- ☐ Atropen
- ☐ Bal in oil
- ☐ calcium disodium
- ☐ Campral
- ☐ catapres
- ☐ Chantix
- ☐ chelating agents
- ☐ Chemet
- ☐ citrovorum factor
- ☐ Cuprimine

| ■ | A |
|---|---|

- ☐ Cyanokit
- ☐ deferoxamine mesylate
- ☐ Desferal
- ☐ Depade
- ☐ Depen
- ☐ Digibind
- ☐ Digoxin
- ☐ dimercaprol
- ☐ disulfiram
- ☐ Edecrin
- ☐ ethacrynic acid
- ☐ flumazenil
- ☐ folinic acid
- ☐ fomepizole
- ☐ Habitrol
- ☐ hydroxocobalamin
- ☐ Isovorin
- ☐ leucovorin rescue
- ☐ Levoleucovorin
- ☐ Liqui-Char
- ☐ magnesium sulfate
- ☐ methylene blue
- ☐ Mucomyst
- ☐ Mucosil
- ☐ nalmefene
- ☐ naloxone
- ☐ naltrexone
- ☐ Narcan
- ☐ NicoDerm CQ
- ☐ Nicorette
- ☐ Penicillamine
- ☐ physostigmine
- ☐ pralidoxime chloride
- ☐ Protopam
- ☐ pyridoxine
- ☐ Revex
- ☐ ReVia
- ☐ Romazicon
- ☐ sodium nitrate
- ☐ sodium thiosulfate
- ☐ Suboxone

| ■ A | ■ A |
|---|---|

- Subutex
- succimer
- Trexan
- universal
- Urolene Blue
- varenicline
- Vivitrex
- Vivitrol
- Wellcovorin

## ■ ANTI-EMETICS

- Aloxi
- Anzemet
- Antivert
- Arrestin
- Atarax
- Benadryl
- Benadryl-D
- Bendectin
- Benzacot
- Bonine
- Bucladin-S
- Cesamet
- chlorpromazine
- Compazine
- Cyclizine
- diphenhydramine
- dolasetron
- Dramamine
- dronabinol
- droperidol
- Elavil
- Emecheck
- Emend
- Emesert
- Emetrol
- fosaprepitant dimeglumine
- Hyoscine
- granisetron
- Kytril
- Little Tummys

- lorazepam
- Marezine
- Marinol
- Maxeran
- meclizine
- Mepergan
- metoclopramide
- midocrine
- MT100
- Nabilone
- Nausetrol
- Nauzene
- Octamide PFS
- Ondansetron
- palonosetron
- perphenazine
- Phenergan
- ProAmatine
- prochlorperazine
- promethazine
- pyridoxine
- Reglan
- Sancuso
- scopolamine
- Sea-Band
- Stemetic
- Tebamide
- thiethylperazine
- Thorazine
- Ticon
- Tigan
- Torecan
- Transderm SCOP
- Triban
- Trilafon
- Tribenzagan
- trimethobenzamide
- Vertigoheel
- Vistaril
- Zofran
- Zontrol

| ■ | A |
|---|---|

| ■ | A |
|---|---|

## ■ ANTI-INFLAMMATORY

- ❑ acetaminophen
- ❑ Acular
- ❑ Advil
- ❑ Aerobid
- ❑ AK-Pred
- ❑ AK-Tate
- ❑ Alka-Butazolidin
- ❑ Alkabutazone
- ❑ Alrex
- ❑ Arlheumet
- ❑ Amersol
- ❑ Anaprox
- ❑ Ansaid
- ❑ Apsifen
- ❑ Arcalyst
- ❑ Arthrotec
- ❑ Asacol
- ❑ Azmacort
- ❑ Azulfidine
- ❑ Baldex
- ❑ balsalazide
- ❑ Beclovent
- ❑ betamethasone
- ❑ betamethasone dipropionate
- ❑ betamethasone valerate
- ❑ Betnesol
- ❑ Bufferin
- ❑ butazolidin
- ❑ CI Inhibitor
- ❑ Cataflam
- ❑ Celebrix
- ❑ certolizumab pegol
- ❑ Cimzia
- ❑ Clinoril
- ❑ Colazal
- ❑ Cordran
- ❑ Cortemed
- ❑ cortisol
- ❑ cortisone
- ❑ Cortisporin

- ❑ Cutivate
- ❑ Cinryze
- ❑ D2E7
- ❑ Dalalone
- ❑ Daypro
- ❑ Decacort
- ❑ Decadron
- ❑ Depo-Medrol
- ❑ DesOwen
- ❑ dexair
- ❑ dexamethasone
- ❑ Dexotic
- ❑ Dexsone
- ❑ diclofenac
- ❑ diflunisal
- ❑ difluprednate
- ❑ Diodex
- ❑ Dipentum
- ❑ Diprolene
- ❑ Disalcid
- ❑ Doan's pills
- ❑ Dolobid
- ❑ Duract
- ❑ Durezol
- ❑ EC-Naprosyn
- ❑ Econopred
- ❑ Eflone
- ❑ enteric aspirin
- ❑ Feldene
- ❑ fenoprofen
- ❑ Flarex
- ❑ flavocoxid
- ❑ floctafenine
- ❑ Flo-Pred
- ❑ Flovent
- ❑ fluorometholone
- ❑ Flur-Op
- ❑ flurbiprofen
- ❑ Haltran
- ❑ hydrocortisone
- ❑ Ibren

| ■ | A | | ■ | A |
|---|---|---|---|---|

- [ ] IBU
- [ ] Ibuprin
- [ ] ibuprofen
- [ ] ibuprofen lysine
- [ ] Ibuprohm
- [ ] Ibu-Tab
- [ ] Indocin
- [ ] indomethacin
- [ ] Inflamase
- [ ] I-Pred
- [ ] ketoprofen
- [ ] ketorolac
- [ ] Lidex
- [ ] Life-Pred
- [ ] Limbrel
- [ ] Lodine
- [ ] Lotemax
- [ ] loteprednol
- [ ] LSAIDS
- [ ] Luxig
- [ ] Lysine
- [ ] Magan
- [ ] magnesium salicylate
- [ ] Magsal
- [ ] Maxidex
- [ ] Meclomen
- [ ] Medipren
- [ ] medrysone
- [ ] meflofenamate
- [ ] mefenamic acid
- [ ] meloxicam
- [ ] mesalamine
- [ ] methylprednisolone
- [ ] Midol
- [ ] Mobic
- [ ] Mobidin
- [ ] Motrin
- [ ] nabumetone
- [ ] Nalfon
- [ ] Naprelan
- [ ] Naprosyn

- [ ] Naproxen
- [ ] NeoDecadron
- [ ] NeoProfen
- [ ] nepafenac
- [ ] Nevanac
- [ ] NSAIDS
- [ ] Nuprin
- [ ] Ocu-Dex
- [ ] Ocufen
- [ ] Ocu-Pred
- [ ] olsalaine
- [ ] Orudis
- [ ] Oruvail
- [ ] oxaprozin
- [ ] Pamprin
- [ ] Paxofen
- [ ] Pedia
- [ ] Pentasa
- [ ] phenylbutazone
- [ ] Phenylone Plus
- [ ] piroxicam
- [ ] Ponstan
- [ ] Ponstel
- [ ] Pred Forte
- [ ] prednisolone
- [ ] Prednisone
- [ ] Profenal
- [ ] Progesic
- [ ] pseudopterosin
- [ ] Psorcon
- [ ] Pulmicort
- [ ] Q-Profen
- [ ] Relafen
- [ ] rilonacept
- [ ] rimexolone
- [ ] rofecoxib
- [ ] Rowasa
- [ ] Rufen
- [ ] salsalate
- [ ] Spersadex
- [ ] Storz-Dexa

| | A | | A |
|---|---|---|---|

- sulfasalazine
- sulindac
- sumatriptan
- Surgam
- Synflex
- tenoxicam
- tiaprofenic acid
- Tilade
- Tobradex
- Tolectin
- Tolmectin
- Topricin
- Toradol
- Trendar
- Traumeel
- Trexima
- Treximet
- triamcinolone
- Trilisate
- Trivaris
- Ultra-Pred
- Ultravate
- Vancenase
- Vanceril
- Vanoxide
- Vexol
- Vicuprofen
- Vioxx
- Voltaren
- Voltarol
- Zeel

## ■ ANTISEPTICS
- Abreva
- Anbesol
- benzalkonium
- Betadine
- Bithionol
- Castellani
- Cepacol
- ChloraPrep

- Chlorseptic
- chlorazene
- chlorhexidine
- Clorpactin
- Diaparene
- Guaiacol
- Halazone
- Herpecin-L
- hexachlorophene
- hexylresorcinol
- Hibiclens
- hydrogen peroxide
- iodine
- isopropyl alcohol
- Kank-A
- merbromin
- Mercurochrome
- Merthiolate
- methylparaben
- Novitra
- Orabase
- Orajel
- oxyguinoline salts
- phenol
- picric acid
- povidone-iodine
- propylparaban
- Proxacol
- pyrogallol
- Releev
- resorcinol
- Tanac
- thimersol
- Thymol
- Zilactin

## ■ ARTHRITIS
- abatacept
- Aclasta
- Acthar
- adalimumab

| A | A |
|---|---|
| ☐ Adlone | ☐ cyclosporine |
| ☐ Aflexa | ☐ D2E7 |
| ☐ Aleve | ☐ DayPro |
| ☐ Alloprim | ☐ Decadron |
| ☐ allopurinol | ☐ Decaject |
| ☐ almotriptan malate | ☐ Delta-Cortef |
| ☐ Amcort | ☐ Deltasone |
| ☐ Anaprox | ☐ Depen |
| ☐ Anturane | ☐ depMedalone |
| ☐ Arava | ☐ Depoject |
| ☐ Aristocort | ☐ Depo-Medrol |
| ☐ Aristospan | ☐ dexamethasone |
| ☐ Arthriten | ☐ Dexasone |
| ☐ Arth-Rx | ☐ Dexone |
| ☐ Ascriptin | ☐ diclofenac |
| ☐ Atolone | ☐ Diflunisal |
| ☐ auranofin | ☐ Diopred |
| ☐ Axert | ☐ Disalcid |
| ☐ Azulfidine | ☐ D-Med injection |
| ☐ BeneJoint | ☐ Dolobid |
| ☐ Benemid | ☐ Duralone |
| ☐ Ben Gay | ☐ Easprin |
| ☐ betamethasone | ☐ EC-Naprosyn |
| ☐ Bextra | ☐ efalizumab |
| ☐ BioLon | ☐ Elaprase |
| ☐ Bufferin | ☐ Enbrel |
| ☐ Cataflam | ☐ etanercept |
| ☐ Celestone | ☐ etodolac |
| ☐ celecoxib | ☐ Feldene |
| ☐ Cel-U-Jec injection | ☐ fenoprofen |
| ☐ Cerebrex | ☐ flavocoxid |
| ☐ chondroitin | ☐ Flexable |
| ☐ Clinoril | ☐ Flexamin |
| ☐ CM Plex | ☐ Flexanew |
| ☐ ColBENEMID | ☐ Flexium |
| ☐ Colchicine | ☐ Folex PFS |
| ☐ COX-2 | ☐ glucosamine |
| ☐ corticotropin | ☐ Haldrone |
| ☐ cortisone | ☐ Hexadrol |
| ☐ Cortone | ☐ H.P. Acthar Gel |
| ☐ Cuprimine | ☐ Humira |

| A | A |
|---|---|
| ☐ Hyalgan | ☐ Pharma Flex |
| ☐ Hyaluronate | ☐ piroxicam |
| ☐ Hydeltra | ☐ Plaqueril |
| ☐ Hydeltrasol | ☐ prednisolone |
| ☐ hydrocortisone | ☐ prednisone |
| ☐ IBU | ☐ Prelone |
| ☐ ibuprofen | ☐ probenecid |
| ☐ idursulfase | ☐ Raptiva |
| ☐ Imuran | ☐ Reclast |
| ☐ Indocin | ☐ Relafen |
| ☐ Inflamase | ☐ Remicade |
| ☐ Infliximab | ☐ Rheumatrex |
| ☐ Kenalog | ☐ Ridaura |
| ☐ ketoprofen | ☐ Rituxan |
| ☐ Kneerelief | ☐ rofecoxib |
| ☐ leflunomide | ☐ Salonpas |
| ☐ Limbrel | ☐ Satogesic |
| ☐ Liquid Pred | ☐ sodium hyaluronate |
| ☐ Lodine | ☐ Solu-Cortef |
| ☐ Lopurin | ☐ Solu-Medrol |
| ☐ Medralone | ☐ sulfinpyrazone |
| ☐ Medrol | ☐ sulindac |
| ☐ methotrexate | ☐ Supartz |
| ☐ methylprednisolone | ☐ Synvisc |
| ☐ Mexate | ☐ Thera-Gesic |
| ☐ Motrin | ☐ ThermaCare |
| ☐ Mono-Gesic | ☐ Tolectin |
| ☐ Myochrysine | ☐ tolmetin sodium |
| ☐ Nalfon | ☐ Triam-A injection |
| ☐ Neoral | ☐ Tri-Kort |
| ☐ Naprelan | ☐ Trilisate |
| ☐ Naprosyn | ☐ Trilog |
| ☐ naproxen | ☐ TripleFlex |
| ☐ Nuflexxa | ☐ Trisoject injection |
| ☐ Orencia | ☐ valdecoxib |
| ☐ Orthovisc | ☐ Vioxx |
| ☐ Orudis | ☐ Voltaren |
| ☐ Oruvail | ☐ Zeel |
| ☐ Osteo Bi-Flex | ☐ zoledronic acid |
| ☐ Pediapred | ☐ Zyloprim |
| ☐ penicillamine | |

| ■ | A |
|---|---|

■ **ASTHMA**
- [ ] Accolate
- [ ] Accuneb
- [ ] Advair Diskus
- [ ] Advair HFA
- [ ] Aerobid
- [ ] AeroCount
- [ ] Aerolate
- [ ] Airet
- [ ] albuterol
- [ ] AllerNaze
- [ ] Allupent
- [ ] Alpha-Proteinase
- [ ] Alvesco
- [ ] aminophylline
- [ ] Ana-Guard
- [ ] Anti-Ige
- [ ] Aralast NP
- [ ] ardeparin sodium
- [ ] arformoterol tartrate
- [ ] Arm-A-Med
- [ ] Asmanex Twisthaler
- [ ] Astepro
- [ ] Asthmalix
- [ ] Asthmahaler
- [ ] AsthmaNefrin
- [ ] Atrovent
- [ ] azelastine
- [ ] Azmacort
- [ ] beclomethasone
- [ ] Beclovent
- [ ] bitolterol mesylate
- [ ] Brethaire
- [ ] Brethine
- [ ] Bricanyl
- [ ] Bronkaid
- [ ] Bronkephrine
- [ ] Bronkosol
- [ ] Brovana
- [ ] butesonide
- [ ] calcitriol

- [ ] Choledyl
- [ ] ciclesonide
- [ ] Combivent
- [ ] cromolyn
- [ ] Decadron Turbinaire
- [ ] Deltasone
- [ ] Dexacort
- [ ] Dey-Dose
- [ ] dexamethasone
- [ ] Duo-Inhaler
- [ ] DuoNeb
- [ ] dyphylline
- [ ] Elixophyllin-KI
- [ ] epinephrine
- [ ] Epi-Pen
- [ ] fenoterol
- [ ] Flonase
- [ ] Flo-Pred
- [ ] Flovent
- [ ] flunisolide
- [ ] fluticasone
- [ ] fluticasone furoate
- [ ] Foradil Aerolizer
- [ ] formoterol fumarate
- [ ] formoterol fumarate dihydrate
- [ ] guaifenesin
- [ ] Qua-Vent
- [ ] hylan
- [ ] Intal Inhaler
- [ ] ipratropium bromide
- [ ] isoetharine
- [ ] isoproterenol
- [ ] Isuprel
- [ ] Lanophyllin
- [ ] Levalbuterol
- [ ] levocetirizine dihydrochloride
- [ ] Maxair Autohaler
- [ ] Medihaler
- [ ] Medaprel
- [ ] Medrol
- [ ] Metaprel

## A

- ☐ metaproterenol
- ☐ methylprednisolone
- ☐ mometasone furoate
- ☐ montelukast
- ☐ Nasacort AQ
- ☐ Nasalcrom
- ☐ Nasalide
- ☐ Nasonex
- ☐ nedocromil
- ☐ Novosalmol
- ☐ olopatadine
- ☐ omalizumab
- ☐ Orapred
- ☐ organidin
- ☐ oxtriphylline
- ☐ Patanase
- ☐ Pedipred
- ☐ Perforomist
- ☐ pirbuterol
- ☐ prednisolone
- ☐ prednisone
- ☐ Prelone
- ☐ Primatene Mist
- ☐ ProAir HFA
- ☐ Prolastin
- ☐ Proventil
- ☐ provocholine
- ☐ Pulmicort Respules
- ☐ Pulmicort Turbhaler
- ☐ Quadrinal
- ☐ Quibron-T/SR
- ☐ QVAR
- ☐ Resogbud
- ☐ salmeterol
- ☐ Serevent
- ☐ Singulair
- ☐ Slo-Bid
- ☐ Spiriva HandiHaler
- ☐ Sus-Phrine
- ☐ Symbicort
- ☐ Theo-24

## B

- ☐ Theo-Dur
- ☐ terbutaline
- ☐ Theochron
- ☐ Theo-Dur
- ☐ theophylline
- ☐ Tilade
- ☐ tiotropium bromide
- ☐ Tornalate
- ☐ T-Phl
- ☐ triamcinolone
- ☐ turbutaline
- ☐ Uni-Dur
- ☐ Uniphyl
- ☐ Vanceril
- ☐ Ventolin
- ☐ Veramyst
- ☐ Volmax
- ☐ Xolair
- ☐ Xopenex
- ☐ Xyzal
- ☐ zafirlukast
- ☐ Zileuton
- ☐ Zyflo
- ☐ Zyflo CR

## ■ BIRTH CONTROL

- ☐ Alesse
- ☐ All-Flex diaphragm
- ☐ Apri
- ☐ Aviane
- ☐ Brevicon
- ☐ BufferGel
- ☐ Conceptrol
- ☐ condom
- ☐ Copper 7
- ☐ Cryselle
- ☐ Cyclessa
- ☐ Dalkan Shield
- ☐ Delfen
- ☐ Demulen
- ☐ Desogen

97

| ■ | B |
|---|---|

- Depo-Provera
- desogestrel
- dinoprostone
- drospirenone
- EMKO
- Empresse
- Enovid
- Estrostep
- ethyl estradiol
- ethynodiol diacetate
- etonogestrel
- Fem-Cap
- Femcon FE
- Femhrt
- GenCept
- Genora
- Implanon
- Jadelle
- Jenest
- Jolivette
- Kariva
- Koro-Flex
- Koromax
- KY-Plus
- Leena
- Levlen
- Levlite
- Levora
- levonorgestrel
- Lippes Loop
- Loestrin
- Loestrin 24 Fe
- Lo/Ovral
- LoSeasonique
- Low-Ogestrel
- Lunelle
- Lybrel
- Marvalon
- medroxyprogesterone
- mestranol
- Microgestin

| ■ | B |
|---|---|

- Micronor
- mifeprex
- mifepristone
- Ministrin
- Min-Ovral
- Mircette
- Mirena
- Modicon
- Mononessa
- Necon
- Nelova
- nonoxynol
- Nora-BE
- Nordette
- norelgestromin
- Norethin
- norethindrone
- Norgestimate
- norgestrel
- Norinyl
- Norplant
- Nor-QD
- Nortrel
- NuvaRing
- Ogestrel
- Ortho-Cept
- Ortho-Creme
- Ortho-Cyclen
- Ortho-Evra
- Ortho-Gynol
- Ortho-Micronor
- Ortho-Novum
- Ortho-Prefest
- Ortho Tri-Cyclen
- Ortho Tri-Cyclen Lo
- Ovcon
- Ovral
- Ovrette
- ParaGard T280
- Plan B
- Portia

## B

- Preven Emergency Kit
- Progestasert
- prostaglandine
- Prostin E2
- Quasense
- Reclipsen
- RU-486
- Seasonale
- Seasonique
- Select
- Semicid
- Solurex
- Sronyx
- Symphasic
- Tilia FE
- Tri-levlin
- Tri-Norinyl
- TriNessa
- Triphasil
- Triquilar
- Tri-Sprintec
- Trivora
- Vasclip
- VCF Film
- Yaz
- Yasmin
- ZenChent
- Zovia

### ■ BLEEDING DISORDERS
- albumin
- BeneFIX
- Ceprotin
- Cera
- cyanocobalamin
- Cycrin
- Dacogen
- DDAVP
- decitabine
- deferasirox
- eculizumab

## C

- Evithrom
- Exjade
- Flexbumin
- Humate-P
- Kogenate
- Kuvan
- Methergine
- methoxy polyethylene glycol-epoetin
- methylergonovine
- Mircera
- Nascobal
- NovoSeven
- Privigen
- Provera
- Recothrom
- sapropterin dihydrochloride
- Soliris
- Stimate
- Thrombin
- Thrombin-JMI
- Xyntha

### ■ CANCER
- Abraxane
- ABVD
- ABX-EGF
- AC
- ACe
- Actiq
- Adriamycin
- Affinitak
- aldesleukin
- alemtuzumab
- Alimta
- Alkeran
- allopurinol
- Aloprim
- Aloxi
- altretamine
- Amen
- A-Methopterin

| ■ C | ■ C |
|---|---|

- [ ] amifostine
- [ ] anastrozole
- [ ] Android
- [ ] Anzemet
- [ ] Aranesp
- [ ] Aredia
- [ ] Arimidex
- [ ] Aromasin
- [ ] Arranon
- [ ] arsenic trioxide
- [ ] asparaginase
- [ ] Avastin
- [ ] AVDP
- [ ] Avinza
- [ ] Avodart
- [ ] azacitidine
- [ ] BACOP
- [ ] Baraclude
- [ ] bendamustine
- [ ] BEP
- [ ] bevacizumab
- [ ] bexarotene
- [ ] Bexxar
- [ ] bicalutamide
- [ ] BiCNU
- [ ] Blenoxane
- [ ] bortezomib
- [ ] Bryostatin
- [ ] Buserelin
- [ ] busulfan
- [ ] Busulfex
- [ ] cabergoline
- [ ] CAF
- [ ] Campath
- [ ] Camptosar
- [ ] CAP
- [ ] capecitabine
- [ ] carboplatin
- [ ] Carbo-Tax
- [ ] carmustine
- [ ] Casamet

- [ ] Casodex
- [ ] CAVE
- [ ] CAV/VAC
- [ ] CC
- [ ] CDDP/VP
- [ ] CDDP/VP-16
- [ ] CCNU
- [ ] CD
- [ ] CeeNu
- [ ] Cera
- [ ] Cerubidine
- [ ] cetuximab
- [ ] CFM
- [ ] CFPT
- [ ] CHL+PRED
- [ ] chlorambucil
- [ ] Chl/VPP
- [ ] CHOP-Bleo
- [ ] CHOP
    - cyclophosphamide
    - doxorubicin
    - vincristine
    - prednisolone
- [ ] cinacalcet
- [ ] CISCA
- [ ] Cisplatin
- [ ] citarabine
- [ ] cladribine
- [ ] CLD-BOMP
- [ ] clofarabine
- [ ] Clolar
- [ ] clonidine
- [ ] CMF
- [ ] CMFP
- [ ] CMV
- [ ] CNOP
- [ ] COB
- [ ] COMLA
- [ ] COMP
- [ ] COP
- [ ] COP-BLAM

|  | C |
|---|---|

- ☐ COPE
- ☐ copegus
- ☐ COPP
- ☐ Cosmegen
- ☐ Cotara
- ☐ Cox-2 inhibitor
- ☐ CP
- ☐ CT
- ☐ CVD
- ☐ CVD+IL 21
- ☐ CVP
- ☐ CVPP
- ☐ Cy/A
- ☐ cyclophosphamide
- ☐ Cytadren
- ☐ Cytosar
- ☐ Cytoxin
- ☐ CYVADIC
- ☐ DA
- ☐ dacarbazine
- ☐ dactinomycin
- ☐ dalteparin
- ☐ dasatinib
- ☐ DAT
- ☐ DAT/DCT
- ☐ daunomycin
- ☐ Daunorubicin
- ☐ DAV
- ☐ Degarelix
- ☐ Depo-Cyt
- ☐ Depo-Provera
- ☐ dexrazoxane
- ☐ DHAP
- ☐ DI
- ☐ Didronel
- ☐ Diflucan
- ☐ DMC
- ☐ Docetaxel
- ☐ Dolasetron
- ☐ Dostinex
- ☐ Doxil

|  | C |
|---|---|

- ☐ doxorubicin
- ☐ Drabinol
- ☐ DTIC-Dome
- ☐ Droxia
- ☐ Duraclon
- ☐ dutasteride
- ☐ EAP
- ☐ EC
- ☐ EDAP
- ☐ ELF
- ☐ Eligard
- ☐ Elitek
- ☐ Ellence
- ☐ Eloxatin
- ☐ Elspar
- ☐ EMA-86
- ☐ Emcyt
- ☐ Emend
- ☐ entecavir
- ☐ EPEG
- ☐ Epirubicin
- ☐ Epogen
- ☐ Epothilone
- ☐ EP/PE
- ☐ epratuzumab
- ☐ Erbitux
- ☐ Ergamisol
- ☐ erlotinib
- ☐ ESHAP
- ☐ Estinyl
- ☐ estramustine
- ☐ Estratab
- ☐ ET-743
- ☐ Ethyol
- ☐ Etopophos
- ☐ etoposide
- ☐ Eulexin
- ☐ EVA
- ☐ Evista
- ☐ exemestane
- ☐ Exisulind

| | C | | | C |
|---|---|---|---|---|

- FAC
- FAM
- FAME
- FAMTX
- Fareston
- Faslodex
- FCE
- F-CL
- fenofibric
- fentanyl citrate
- Fentora
- filgrastim
- Fle
- FMV
- floxuridine
- Fludara
- fludarabine
- flutamide
- fosaprepitant dimeglumine
- Fragmin
- FUDR
- FU/LV
- fulvestrant
- Gardasil
- gemcitabine
- gemcitabine-Cis
- gemtuzumab
- Gemzar
- Gleevec
- Gliadel
- goserelin
- granisetron
- HDMGTX
- HDMTX
- HepaGam B
- Herceptin
- Hexalen
- HI-CDAZE
- Hycamtin
- Hydrea
- hydroxurea

- ICE
- Idamycin
- idarubicin
- IDMTX/6-MP
- IE
- IFEX
- ifosfamide
- IFoVP
- IMF
- imatinib
- IMVP-16
- interferon
- Intron A
- Iressa
- irinotecan
- Isovorin
- ixabepilone
- Ixempra
- Kepivance
- Kytril
- lanreotide acetate
- lapatinib
- LDAC
- lenalidomide
- Leucovorin
- Leukeran
- Leukine
- leuprolide
- Leustatin
- Levoleucovorin
- Lexidronam
- livamisole
- lomustine
- Lupron
- L-VAM
- Lysodren
- MACOP-B
- MAID
- Marinol
- Matulane
- m-BACOD

| C | C |
|---|---|

- M-BACOS
- MC
- mechlorethamine
- medroxyprogesterone
- Megace
- melphalan
- mercapturine
- mesna
- Mesnex
- methotrexate
- methyl aminolevulinate
- Metvixia
- micafungin
- MINE
- MINE-ESHAP
- Miraluma test
- Mithricin
- mitomycin
- mitoxantrone
- MM
- MMC
- MOBP
- MOP
- MOPP/ABV Hybrid
- MOPP
- MP
- m-PFL
- MTX
- MTX-CDDPAdr
- MTX/6-MP
- MTX/6-MP/VP
- Mustargen
- Mutamycin
- MV
- MVAC
- MVPP
- Mycamine
- Myleran
- Mylotarg
- Nabilone
- Navelbine

- nelarabine
- Neovastat
- Neulasta
- Neupogen
- Nexavar
- NFL
- Nilandron
- nilotinib
- nilutamide
- Nipent
- Nolvadex
- Novantrone
- NOVP
- Noxafil
- Nplate
- Nuvion
- octreotide
- Oncaspar
- Oncolym
- Oncovin
- On-Q
- Ontak
- OPA
- OPPA
- OraVescent Fentanyl
- Orzel
- OvaRex
- oxaliplatin
- ozogamicin
- PAC
- paclitaxel
- palifermin
- pamidronate
- panitumumab
- papillomavirus
- Paraplatin
- PC
- PCV
- pegaspargase
- pegfilgrastim
- PEG-Intron

| | C |
|---|---|

- ❑ pemetrexed
- ❑ PFL
- ❑ PFL+IFN
- ❑ Photofrin
- ❑ pilocarpine
- ❑ placlitaxel
- ❑ Platinol
- ❑ Plenaxis
- ❑ plicamycin
- ❑ POC
- ❑ POMP
-   Purinethol
-   Oncovin
-   Methotrexate
-   Prednisone
- ❑ porfimer sodium
- ❑ posaconazole
- ❑ Procrit
- ❑ Proleukin
- ❑ Pro-MACE-CytaBOM
- ❑ Purinethol
- ❑ Pt-EU
- ❑ PTK 787
- ❑ Pt/VM
- ❑ PVB
- ❑ PVD
- ❑ PVDA
- ❑ Quadramet
- ❑ quadrivalent
- ❑ Raloxifene
- ❑ rasburicase
- ❑ rebetol
- ❑ Revimid
- ❑ Revlimid
- ❑ ribasphere
- ❑ Ribavirin
- ❑ Rituxan
- ❑ rituximab
- ❑ Roferon
- ❑ romiplostim
- ❑ Rubex

| | C |
|---|---|

- ❑ Salagen
- ❑ Sancuso
- ❑ Sandostatin
- ❑ sargramostim
- ❑ Sativex
- ❑ Sclerosol
- ❑ Sensipar
- ❑ Sequential Dox-CMF
- ❑ SMF
- ❑ Soltamox
- ❑ Somatuline Autogel
- ❑ Somatuline Depot
- ❑ sorafenib
- ❑ Sprycel
- ❑ Stanford V
- ❑ streptozocin
- ❑ Sugen
- ❑ sunitinib
- ❑ Suprefact
- ❑ Sutent
- ❑ SU-101
- ❑ SU 11248
- ❑ Tabloid
- ❑ Tamoxifen
- ❑ Tarceva
- ❑ Targretin
- ❑ Tasigna
- ❑ Taxol
- ❑ Taxotere
- ❑ telbivudine
- ❑ temsirolimus
- ❑ teniposide
- ❑ tenofovir disoproxil fumarate
- ❑ Teslac
- ❑ testolactone
- ❑ Testred
- ❑ ThermoDox
- ❑ TheraCys
- ❑ thioguanine
- ❑ Thioplex
- ❑ thiotepa

| ■ | C |
|---|---|

- Thyrogen
- ThyroShield
- TICE BCG
- TIP
- TIT
- Topo/CTX
- topotecan
- Toposar
- toremifene citrate
- Torisel
- tositumomab
- Totect
- tranylcypromine sulfate
- Treanda
- Trelstar Depot
- Trelstar LA
- tretinoin
- Trexall
- Trilipix
- Trisenox
- Tykerb
- Tyzeka
- Uvadex
- VAB VI
- VAC
- VACAdr
- VACAdr-IfoVP
- VAD
- VAdrC
- Valstar
- Vancomycin
- VATH
- VBAP
- VBMCP
- VBP
- VCAP
- Vectibix
- Velban
- Velcade
- VePesid
- Vesanoid

| ■ | C |
|---|---|

- Vidaza
- vinblastine
- vincristine
- vinorelbine
- Vinorelbine-Cis
- VIP
- VIP [Einhorn]
- Viread
- vorinostat
- VP
- Vumon
- Xcytrin
- Xeloda
- Zevalin
- Zofran
- Zoladex
- Zyloprim
- Zanosar
- Zinecard
- Zolinza

## ■ CARDIOLOGY

- Abbokinase
- abciximab
- Accupril
- Accuretic
- Aceon
- ACOVA
- Activase
- Adalat
- Adenocard
- Adenoscan
- adenosine
- Advicor
- Afeditab CR
- Aggrastat
- Aggrenox
- Agrylin
- Aldactazide
- Aldactone
- Aldoclor

| | **C** | | | **C** |
|---|---|---|---|---|

- ❑ Aldomet
- ❑ Aldoril
- ❑ aliskiren
- ❑ Altace
- ❑ alteplase
- ❑ Altoprev
- ❑ ambrisentan
- ❑ amiloride
- ❑ Aminohippurate
- ❑ amiodarone
- ❑ amlodipine
- ❑ amlodipine besylate
- ❑ Ana-Kit
- ❑ Ancrod
- ❑ Ancobon
- ❑ Angiomax
- ❑ Anhydron
- ❑ anisindione
- ❑ Antara
- ❑ ApoA-1
- ❑ ApoA-1 Milano
- ❑ aprotinin
- ❑ Aquatensen
- ❑ Aramine
- ❑ Aranesp
- ❑ Argatroban
- ❑ Arixtra
- ❑ Atacand
- ❑ Atenolol
- ❑ Atorvastatin
- ❑ Atromid-S
- ❑ Avalide
- ❑ Avapro
- ❑ Azor
- ❑ Baycol
- ❑ Benazepril
- ❑ bendroflumethiazide
- ❑ Benicar
- ❑ benzthiazide
- ❑ bepridil
- ❑ Betapace

- ❑ BiDil
- ❑ BioZ monitor
- ❑ bivalirudin
- ❑ Blocadren
- ❑ Brevibloc
- ❑ Bumetanide
- ❑ Bystolic
- ❑ Caduet
- ❑ candesartan cilexetil
- ❑ Calan
- ❑ Captopen
- ❑ Captopril
- ❑ Captozide
- ❑ Cardene
- ❑ Cardio Essentials
- ❑ CardioGen 82
- ❑ cardioplegic solution
- ❑ Cardioquin
- ❑ CardioTec Kit
- ❑ Cardizem
- ❑ Cardura
- ❑ Cartia XT
- ❑ Cartrol
- ❑ Carvedilol
- ❑ Catapres
- ❑ Catapres-TTS
- ❑ Cathflo Activase
- ❑ cerivastatin
- ❑ chlorothiazide
- ❑ chlorthalidone
- ❑ cholestyramine
- ❑ cilostazol
- ❑ clevidipine
- ❑ Cleviprex
- ❑ clofibrate
- ❑ clopidogrel
- ❑ Clorpres-TTS
- ❑ Colestid
- ❑ colestipol
- ❑ colesevelam
- ❑ Combipres

| C | C |
|---|---|

- Cordarone
- Coreg
- Coricidin HBP
- Covera-HS
- Corlopam
- Corvert
- Corzide
- Cozaar
- CP-529
- Crestor
- cyclothiazide
- Cypher stent
- dalteparin
- danaparoid
- Daramode
- Daranide
- Darbepoetin Alfa
- Demadex
- Demser
- Deponit
- dibenzyline
- dichlorphenamide
- Digibind
- Digitek
- digoxin
- Dilacor XR
- Diltazem
- Diovan
- dipyridamole
- Diucardin
- Diuchlor
- Diulo
- Diupres
- Diuril
- dobutamine
- Dobutrex
- dofetilide
- Doxazosin
- Durectic
- Dyazide
- Dyrenium

- Ecotrin
- eculizumab
- Edecrine
- Eminase
- enalapril maleate
- Encainide
- Endeavor
- Enduron
- Enkaid
- enoxaparin
- Epi-Pen
- Epoprostenol
- eprosartan mesylate
- eptifibatide
- erythropoietin
- Esidrix
- Esimil
- esmolol
- ethacrynate sodium
- ethacrynic
- ethaverine
- Ethavex-100
- Ethmozine
- Exanta
- Exforge
- Exna
- ezetimibe
- felodipine
- fenofibrate
- fenofibric
- Fenoglide
- flecainide
- Flolan
- flucytosine
- Fluidex
- fluvastatin
- fondaparinux
- Fragmin
- Furosemide
- gemfibrozil
- Genabid

| ■ C | ■ C |
|---|---|
| ❑ Glucagon | ❑ Lanoxin |
| ❑ glucose | ❑ Lasix |
| ❑ Glutose | ❑ lercanidipine |
| ❑ glyceryl trinitrate | ❑ Lescol |
| ❑ Guanabenz | ❑ Letairis |
| ❑ Guanadrel | ❑ Levatol |
| ❑ Guanethidine | ❑ Levostatin |
| ❑ guanfacine | ❑ Lexiscan |
| ❑ Halfprin | ❑ Lexxel |
| ❑ Hespan | ❑ Lipitor |
| ❑ hetastarch | ❑ LoCholest |
| ❑ hydralazine hydrochloride | ❑ Lofibra |
| ❑ Hydrex | ❑ Lopid |
| ❑ hydrochlorothiazide | ❑ Lorelco |
| ❑ Hydro-D | ❑ losartan |
| ❑ HydroDIURIL | ❑ Lotrel |
| ❑ hydroflumethiazide | ❑ lovastatin |
| ❑ Hydromox | ❑ Lovaza |
| ❑ Hylorel | ❑ Lovenox |
| ❑ Hyperstat | ❑ Mavik |
| ❑ Hytrin | ❑ Maxzide |
| ❑ Hyzaar | ❑ Merci Retreiver |
| ❑ ibutilide | ❑ Metahydrin |
| ❑ Imdur | ❑ methyclothiazide |
| ❑ Indapamide | ❑ metolazone |
| ❑ Inderal | ❑ metoprolol |
| ❑ Inderide | ❑ Mevacor |
| ❑ Innohep | ❑ Mexitil |
| ❑ Integrilin | ❑ micronized colestipol |
| ❑ Inversine | ❑ Microzide |
| ❑ irbesartan | ❑ Midamor |
| ❑ ISMO | ❑ Midodrine |
| ❑ Ismelin | ❑ milrinone |
| ❑ Isoptin SR | ❑ Minipress |
| ❑ Isordil | ❑ Minizide |
| ❑ isosorbide dinitrate | ❑ Moduretic |
| ❑ Isoxsuprine | ❑ Monoket |
| ❑ Kabikinase | ❑ Monopril |
| ❑ Kerlone | ❑ moricizine |
| ❑ Lanoxican | ❑ Mykrox |
| ❑ Lanoxicaps | ❑ Nadolol |

| ■ C | ■ C |
|---|---|
| ❑ Natrecor | ❑ Plendil |
| ❑ nebivolol | ❑ Pletal |
| ❑ Neo-Codema | ❑ Plavix |
| ❑ nesiritide | ❑ Plegisol |
| ❑ Nexterone | ❑ polythiazide |
| ❑ niacin | ❑ Posicor |
| ❑ nicardipine | ❑ Pravachol |
| ❑ Niaspan | ❑ pravastatin |
| ❑ Nicolar | ❑ Pravigard |
| ❑ nifedipine | ❑ Primacor |
| ❑ nimodipine | ❑ Prinivil |
| ❑ Nimotop | ❑ ProAmatine |
| ❑ Nisoldipine | ❑ procainamide |
| ❑ Nitro-Bid | ❑ Procanbid |
| ❑ Nitro-Derm | ❑ Procardia |
| ❑ Nitrodisc | ❑ Procrit Epoetin Alfa |
| ❑ Nitro-Dur | ❑ Proflavanol |
| ❑ nitroglycerin | ❑ propafenone |
| ❑ NitroMist | ❑ propranolol |
| ❑ Nitrostat | ❑ Prostin VR |
| ❑ Nitrolingual | ❑ protamine sulfate |
| ❑ Normiflo | ❑ Questran |
| ❑ Normodyne | ❑ quinethazone |
| ❑ Norpace | ❑ Quinidex |
| ❑ Norvasc | ❑ quinidine |
| ❑ Novo-Hydrazide | ❑ ranolazine |
| ❑ Novo-Thalidone | ❑ Ranexa |
| ❑ Odrinil | ❑ Rasilez |
| ❑ olmesartan | ❑ regadenoson |
| ❑ olmesartan Medoxomil | ❑ Remodulin |
| ❑ Omacor | ❑ Renese |
| ❑ Oretic | ❑ ReoPro |
| ❑ Orgaran | ❑ Retavase |
| ❑ Pacerone | ❑ Reteplase |
| ❑ papaverine | ❑ Revatio |
| ❑ Pavabid | ❑ rosuvastatin |
| ❑ Pavatine | ❑ Rythmol |
| ❑ pentoxifylline | ❑ Saluron |
| ❑ Persantine | ❑ Sectral |
| ❑ phenylephrine | ❑ Ser-Ap-Es |
| ❑ phytosterol blocker | ❑ sildenafil citrate |

| | C |
|---|---|

- Simcor
- simvastatin
- sodium edecrin
- sodium nitroprusside
- Soliris
- Sorbitrate
- sotalol
- spironolactone
- stanozolol
- Streptase
- Streptokinase
- Sular
- Sunril
- Tamocor
- Tarka
- Teczem
- Tekturna
- telmisartan
- tenecteplase
- Tenex
- Tenoretic
- Tenormin
- Teveten
- Thalitone
- Tiazac
- Ticlid
- Tikosyn
- ticlopidine
- Tilosyn
- tinzaparin
- tirofaban
- TNKase
- tocainide
- Tonocard
- Toprol-XL
- torcetrapib
- torsemide
- TPA
- trandolapril
- Trasylol
- Trental

| | C |
|---|---|

- Treprostinil
- triamterene
- trichlormethiazide
- TriCor
- Triglide
- Trilipix
- UK-68-798
- Unvasc
- Uniretic
- Uridon
- Urozide
- valsartan
- Vanlev
- Vascor
- Vaseretic
- Vasodilan
- Vasotec
- Vasoxyl
- Ventavis
- verapamil
- Verelan
- Vytorin
- WelChol
- Winstrol
- Wytensin
- Xience
- ximelagatran
- Zaroxolyn
- Zebeta
- Zestoretic
- Zestril
- Zetia
- Ziac
- Zinecard
- Zocor
- Zotarolimus

## ■ COLD+COUGH

- acetaminophen
- Actifed
- Advil

| ■ C | ■ C |
|-----|-----|
| ☐ Alacor DM Syrup | ☐ Clarinex |
| ☐ Afrin | ☐ Clarinex-D |
| ☐ Alfa CF | ☐ Codeprex |
| ☐ Allegra | ☐ Codiclear |
| ☐ Allegra-D | ☐ Coldcalm |
| ☐ AllerNaze | ☐ Cold-EEZE |
| ☐ Allerx | ☐ Comhist |
| ☐ Allfen | ☐ Comtrex |
| ☐ Aleve | ☐ Congess |
| ☐ Ambifed | ☐ Contac |
| ☐ Amerifed | ☐ Contac-D |
| ☐ Anatuss | ☐ Coricidin |
| ☐ Arco-Lase | ☐ Coricidin HBP |
| ☐ Ascriptin | ☐ Creomulsion |
| ☐ astemizole | ☐ Cromolyn |
| ☐ Astepro | ☐ DayQuil |
| ☐ Atrohist | ☐ Decacort |
| ☐ Avelox | ☐ Deconamine |
| ☐ Ayr | ☐ Deconsal |
| ☐ azelastine | ☐ Deconsat |
| ☐ Balamine | ☐ Delsym |
| ☐ Baltussin | ☐ Desloratadine |
| ☐ Benadryl | ☐ Despec |
| ☐ Benadryl-D | ☐ dexamethasone |
| ☐ Benzedrex | ☐ dexbrompheniramine |
| ☐ benzonatate | ☐ dextromethorphan |
| ☐ Boiron | ☐ Diabe-Tuss DM |
| ☐ Boostrix | ☐ Dimetane |
| ☐ Boroleum | ☐ Dimetapp |
| ☐ Bromfed | ☐ Diphedryl |
| ☐ brompheniramine | ☐ Dristan |
| ☐ Brontex | ☐ Drixoral |
| ☐ Bufferin | ☐ Duratex |
| ☐ Cantil | ☐ Duratuss |
| ☐ cetirizine | ☐ Echinacea |
| ☐ Cheracol | ☐ Emergen-C |
| ☐ chlorpheniramine | ☐ Entex |
| ☐ chlorpheniramine polistirex | ☐ ENTSOL |
| ☐ Chlor-Trimeton | ☐ Excedrin |
| ☐ ciclesonide | ☐ Exgest |
| ☐ Claritin | ☐ Extendryl |

|  | C |
|--|---|

- Fedahist
- fexofenadine
- glyceryl guaiacolate
- Guaifed
- guaifenesin
- Guaimax
- Halotussin
- Hismanal
- Histussin
- Humibid
- hydrocodone
- Inspire
- Isoclor
- Liquibid
- Lufyllin
- Maxidone
- moxifloxacin
- Mucinex
- Mucinex Mini-Melts
- Nasacort AQ
- NasalCrom
- Nasonex
- Neo-Synephrine
- Nostrilla
- Nytol
- Nyquill
- Ocean
- olopatadine
- Omnaris
- Oscillo
- Oscillococcin
- Organidin
- Ornex
- Otrivin
- oxymetazoline
- Patanase
- PediaCare
- Pediacof
- Phenergan
- phenylephrine
- Picovir

- pleconaril
- Profen IB
- Prometh
- promethazine
- pseudoephedrine
- Quadrinal
- Quibron
- Rescon
- Robitussin
- Rondec
- Rynatan
- Rynatuss
- Rhinosyn
- Similasan
- Sine-Off
- Sinex
- SinoFresh
- Sinulin
- Sinupan
- Sinutab
- Sominex
- Sudafed
- Syn-Rx
- Tessalon
- Theraflu
- triamcinolone
- Triaminic
- Triaminic Softchews
- Triaminicin
- Trinalin
- Tussagesic
- Tussend
- Tussin
- Tussionex Pennkinetic
- Tussi-Organidin DM
- Unisom
- Vicks
- Vicks 44D
- Vicks 44E
- Vicks Casero
- Vicks DayQuil

**D**

- Vicks Nyquil
- Vicks Sinex
- Vicks VapoRub
- Vicks VapoSteam
- XL-3
- xylometazoline
- Zicam
- Zyrtec

# ■ DERMATOLOGY

- 8-Mop
- Abreva
- Acanya
- acitretin
- Accutane
- Acitretin
- Aclovate
- Acticin
- Actinex
- Actiza
- Aclovate
- acyclovir
- Aczone
- adapalene
- Aftate
- Alferon
- Aldara
- alitretinoin
- allium cepa
- Alpha-Hydroxy
- Altabax
- Alti-Acyclovir
- Alustra
- amcinonide
- Amevive
- aminolevulinic acid
- aminophylline
- AmLactin AP
- AmLactin XL
- Anbesol
- anidulafungin

**D**

- Anxanil
- anthralin
- Appearex
- Aquanil
- Aquaphor
- Artecoll
- Artefill
- Atrac-Tain
- Aristocort
- Aristospan
- Artiss
- Atarax
- Atopiclair
- Atralin
- A/T/S
- Avage
- AVC
- Aveeno
- Avirax
- Avita
- Avobenzone
- azelaic acid
- Azelex
- Bactine
- Band-Aid Scar Healing
- Benadryl
- Benadryl-D
- Benoquin
- bentoquatam
- Benzac
- Benzaclin
- Benzamycin
- Benziq
- benzoyl peroxide
- betamethasone
- betamethasone dipropionate
- betamethasone valerate
- bichloracetic acid Kahlenberg
- Biore
- Brevoxyl
- butenafine

113

| ■ D | ■ D |
|-----|-----|
| ❏ Caladryl | ❏ Cortone |
| ❏ CalaGel | ❏ Cortizone-10 |
| ❏ calamine | ❏ CosmoDerm |
| ❏ calcipotriene | ❏ CosmoPlast |
| ❏ Caldesene | ❏ cromolyn sodium |
| ❏ Campho-Phenique | ❏ crotamiton |
| ❏ Capex | ❏ Curad Scar Therapy |
| ❏ capryloyl glycine | ❏ Curel |
| ❏ Captique | ❏ Cutivate |
| ❏ Carac cream | ❏ Cyclocort |
| ❏ Carlesta | ❏ cyclosporine |
| ❏ Carmex | ❏ Dagenan |
| ❏ Cellulean | ❏ dapsone |
| ❏ Cetaphil lotion | ❏ Decaspray |
| ❏ ChapStick | ❏ Denavir |
| ❏ Cica-Care | ❏ Denorex |
| ❏ ciclopirox olamine | ❏ Dermarest |
| ❏ Cinryze | ❏ DermaSmoothe |
| ❏ Claripel | ❏ Dermatop |
| ❏ Clean & Clear | ❏ Desenex |
| ❏ Clearasil | ❏ Desitin |
| ❏ Clear Away | ❏ Desonate |
| ❏ Clenia | ❏ desonide |
| ❏ Cleocin | ❏ Desowen |
| ❏ Clinac | ❏ desoxymetasone |
| ❏ Clindagel | ❏ Desquam |
| ❏ clindamycin | ❏ dexamethasone |
| ❏ clindamycin hydrochloride | ❏ DHS tar shampoo |
| ❏ Clioquinol | ❏ Diabet-X |
| ❏ clobetasol propionate | ❏ Differin |
| ❏ Clobevate | ❏ diflorasone |
| ❏ Clobex | ❏ Diprolene |
| ❏ clotrimazole | ❏ Diprosone |
| ❏ Collagenase | ❏ Dithrocreme |
| ❏ Compound W | ❏ Domeboro |
| ❏ Condylox | ❏ Dovonex |
| ❏ Cordran | ❏ doxepin |
| ❏ Cormax | ❏ Duac |
| ❏ Cortaid | ❏ DuoFilm |
| ❏ cortisone | ❏ efalizumab |
| ❏ Cortisporin | ❏ Eldopaque |

| ■ D | ■ D |
|---|---|
| ❑ Eldoquin | ❑ griseofulvin |
| ❑ Eletone cream | ❑ GRIS-PEG |
| ❑ Elevess | ❑ Grifulvin |
| ❑ Elidel | ❑ halcinonide |
| ❑ Elimite | ❑ halobetasol |
| ❑ Elocon | ❑ Halog |
| ❑ Emgel | ❑ Head & Shoulders |
| ❑ Enydrial | ❑ Herpecin-L |
| ❑ Epiduo | ❑ hydrocortisone |
| ❑ Ertaczo | ❑ Hydrocortone |
| ❑ Erycette | ❑ hydroquinone |
| ❑ Erythra-Derm | ❑ hydroxyzine pamoate |
| ❑ erythromycin ethylsuccinate | ❑ Hylaform |
| ❑ esterase | ❑ hyaluronic acid |
| ❑ Estrostep | ❑ Hytone |
| ❑ ETS-2 % | ❑ imidazole |
| ❑ Eucerin | ❑ imiquimod |
| ❑ Eurex | ❑ interferon alfa |
| ❑ Excelderm | ❑ Invanz |
| ❑ Evoclin | ❑ iodoquinol |
| ❑ Evolence | ❑ Ionil-T |
| ❑ Extina | ❑ Iontophoretic |
| ❑ Finacea | ❑ isotretinoin |
| ❑ Finevin | ❑ Ivarest |
| ❑ fluocinolone | ❑ IvyBLock |
| ❑ Fluoroplex | ❑ Ivy-Dry |
| ❑ fluorouracil | ❑ IvyStat! |
| ❑ flurandrenolide | ❑ Juvederm |
| ❑ fluticasone | ❑ Kank-A |
| ❑ Formadon | ❑ ketoconazole |
| ❑ formaldehyde | ❑ Klaron |
| ❑ Fototar | ❑ KP Duty |
| ❑ Fulvicin | ❑ kunecatechins |
| ❑ Fungi Care | ❑ L.M.X.4 cream |
| ❑ Fungi Clear | ❑ L.M.X.5 cream |
| ❑ Garamycin | ❑ Lac-Hydrin |
| ❑ GentleWave | ❑ Laclotion |
| ❑ glycerin | ❑ Lamisil |
| ❑ glycyrrhetinic acid | ❑ Lanacane |
| ❑ Glyquin | ❑ lanolin |
| ❑ Gold Bond | ❑ Lazerformaldehyde |

| ■ | D | ■ | D |
|---|---|---|---|

- ❑ levocetirizine dihydrochloride
- ❑ Levulan Kerastick
- ❑ Lidex
- ❑ LidoSite
- ❑ Lindane lotion
- ❑ Loprox
- ❑ L'Oreal
- ❑ Lotrimin
- ❑ Lotrisone
- ❑ Lubriderm
- ❑ Lustro
- ❑ Luxiq
- ❑ Malathion
- ❑ Masoprocol
- ❑ Maxiflor
- ❑ Mederma
- ❑ Melanax
- ❑ meloxicam
- ❑ Mentadil
- ❑ Mentax
- ❑ methoxsalen
- ❑ methyl aminolevulinate
- ❑ Metrocream
- ❑ Metrogel
- ❑ metronidazole cream
- ❑ Metvixia
- ❑ Micanol
- ❑ Micatin
- ❑ miconazole
- ❑ Mimyx
- ❑ Mintezol
- ❑ Miracle of Aloe Miracure
- ❑ Mobic
- ❑ Mobisyl
- ❑ Moisturel
- ❑ mometasone
- ❑ Monistat-Derm
- ❑ monobenzone
- ❑ Multipax
- ❑ Mycostatin
- ❑ naftifine

- ❑ Naftin
- ❑ Neoral
- ❑ Neosporin
- ❑ Neutrogena
- ❑ Nicomide
- ❑ nicotinamide
- ❑ Nix Crème
- ❑ Nizoral A-D
- ❑ Noritate
- ❑ Novitra
- ❑ Novo-Hydroxyzin
- ❑ Noxzema
- ❑ NuFill
- ❑ Nystatin
- ❑ Occusal-HP
- ❑ Olay
- ❑ Olay Regenerist
- ❑ Olux Foam
- ❑ Olux-E Foam
- ❑ Orabase
- ❑ Oracea
- ❑ Orajel
- ❑ Ovide
- ❑ Oxy
- ❑ Oxyconazole
- ❑ Oxsoralen-Ultra
- ❑ Oxystat
- ❑ Paddock Podifilox
- ❑ Pandel
- ❑ PanOxyl
- ❑ Panretin gel
- ❑ penciclovir
- ❑ Perlane
- ❑ pHisoderm
- ❑ pHisoHex
- ❑ pimecorlimus
- ❑ Pin-Rid
- ❑ Polytar shampoo
- ❑ Prelone
- ❑ Podocon
- ❑ podofilox

|  | **D** |  |  | **D** |
|---|---|---|---|---|

- ❑ Polyphenon E
- ❑ Pramegel
- ❑ Pramosone
- ❑ prednisolone
- ❑ Preparation H
- ❑ Pro-Clerz
- ❑ Prograniq
- ❑ Prosacea
- ❑ Prudoxin
- ❑ Psorcon cream
- ❑ Psoriasin gel
- ❑ pyrantel pamoate
- ❑ Radiance
- ❑ Radiesse
- ❑ Raptiva
- ❑ Releev
- ❑ Renova
- ❑ Restylane
- ❑ retapamulin
- ❑ Retina-A-Micro
- ❑ Rid Lice
- ❑ Roc
- ❑ Rosac wash
- ❑ Salac
- ❑ salicylic acid
- ❑ Santyl
- ❑ Scalpicin
- ❑ Sclerosol intrapleural
- ❑ Sculptra
- ❑ Sebazole
- ❑ Sebulex
- ❑ Selsun
- ❑ SERPACWA
- ❑ sertaconazole
- ❑ shea butter
- ❑ skinMilk
- ❑ sodium sulfacetamide
- ❑ Solage
- ❑ Solarcaine
- ❑ Solodyn
- ❑ Soriatane

- ❑ Spenco 2nd Skin Scar
- ❑ St. Ives
- ❑ Stridex
- ❑ StriVectin-HS
- ❑ StriVectin-SD
- ❑ sulconazole
- ❑ Sulfacet
- ❑ sulfapyridine
- ❑ Swabplus
- ❑ Synalar
- ❑ Synemol
- ❑ Taclonex
- ❑ Tanac
- ❑ Tavist
- ❑ tazarotene gel
- ❑ Tazorac
- ❑ Temovate
- ❑ terbinafine
- ❑ thalidomide
- ❑ Thalomid
- ❑ Thermage
- ❑ Thiobendazole
- ❑ tigecycline
- ❑ Tinactin
- ❑ Tinamed
- ❑ Tineacide
- ❑ Topicort
- ❑ tretinoin
- ❑ triamcinolone
- ❑ Triaz
- ❑ Tridesilon
- ❑ Tri-Luma
- ❑ trioxsalen
- ❑ Trisoralen
- ❑ T-Stat
- ❑ Tucks
- ❑ Tygacil
- ❑ Ultravate
- ❑ valacyclovir
- ❑ Valtrex
- ❑ Vanos

| ■ | D |
|---|---|

- ❏ Vanoxide-HC lotion
- ❏ Vaseline
- ❏ Verdeso
- ❏ Veregen
- ❏ Vioform
- ❏ Vistaril
- ❏ Vytone cream
- ❏ Xanelim
- ❏ Xenaderm
- ❏ Xolegel
- ❏ Xyzal
- ❏ Yaz
- ❏ ZAPZYT
- ❏ Zeasorb
- ❏ Zetar Emulsion
- ❏ Ziana
- ❏ Zilactin
- ❏ Zonalon

## ■ DIABETES

- ❏ acarbose
- ❏ acetohexamide
- ❏ ACTOplus met
- ❏ Actos
- ❏ Amaryl
- ❏ Apidra
- ❏ Ascensia Breeze
- ❏ Aspart
- ❏ atorvastatin
- ❏ Avandaryl
- ❏ Avandia
- ❏ Breeze2
- ❏ Byetta
- ❏ chlorpropamide
- ❏ colesevelam
- ❏ Cymbalta
- ❏ DDAVP
- ❏ detemir
- ❏ DiaBeta
- ❏ Diabinese
- ❏ Diazoxide

| ■ | D |
|---|---|

- ❏ Duetact
- ❏ duloxetine
- ❏ Euglucon
- ❏ Exenatide
- ❏ exendin-4
- ❏ Exubera
- ❏ Fortamet
- ❏ Gen-Glybe
- ❏ Glargine
- ❏ glimepiride
- ❏ glipizide
- ❏ Glucagen
- ❏ Glucagon
- ❏ Glucamide
- ❏ Glucophage
- ❏ Glucotrol
- ❏ Glucovance
- ❏ glulisine
- ❏ Glumetza
- ❏ glyburide
- ❏ Glynase
- ❏ Glynase Prestab
- ❏ Glyset
- ❏ Humalog pen and Kwikpen
- ❏ Humulin 50/50
- ❏ Humulin 70/30
- ❏ Humulin N
- ❏ Humulin R
- ❏ Iletin II, Lente
- ❏ Iletin Ii, NPH
- ❏ Increlex
- ❏ Insulatard
- ❏ insulin
- ❏ insulin aspart protamine
- ❏ insulin detemir
- ❏ insulin glargine
- ❏ insulin glulisine
- ❏ insulin human
- ❏ insulin lispro
- ❏ insulin lispro protamine
- ❏ iPlex

| D |
|---|

- ❏ Janumet
- ❏ Januvia
- ❏ Lantus
- ❏ Lantus SoloStar
- ❏ Lente
- ❏ Lente Iletin II
- ❏ Levemir
- ❏ Lipitor
- ❏ Lispro
- ❏ Lyrica
- ❏ mecasermin
- ❏ Medi-Glybe
- ❏ meglitinide
- ❏ metformin
- ❏ Micronase
- ❏ miglitol
- ❏ Mixtard
- ❏ Nataglinide
- ❏ Novo-Butamide
- ❏ Novo-Glyburide
- ❏ Novolin
- ❏ Novolin N PenFill
- ❏ NovolinPen
- ❏ NovoLog
- ❏ NovoPen
- ❏ NPH Iletin
- ❏ NPH Pork Isophane
- ❏ Nu-Glyburide
- ❏ Orinase
- ❏ pioglitazone
- ❏ pramlintide
- ❏ PrandiMet
- ❏ Prandin
- ❏ Precose
- ❏ pregabalin
- ❏ Proglycem
- ❏ Protamine Zinc
- ❏ PZI
- ❏ Rezulin
- ❏ repaglinide
- ❏ rosiglitazone

| D |
|---|

- ❏ Semilente Iletin
- ❏ sitagliptin
- ❏ SomatoKine
- ❏ Starlix
- ❏ Symlin
- ❏ sulfonylurea
- ❏ Tolamide
- ❏ tolazamide
- ❏ tolbutamide
- ❏ Tolinase
- ❏ Ultralente
- ❏ Troglitazone
- ❏ Velosulin
- ❏ WelChol

## ■ DIARRHEA

- ❏ Alinia
- ❏ alosetron
- ❏ Amitiza
- ❏ cantil
- ❏ Charcocaps
- ❏ Citrucel
- ❏ clindamycin
- ❏ Clindet
- ❏ Coly-Mycin
- ❏ Dia-Quel
- ❏ Diastay
- ❏ Diastop
- ❏ difenoxin
- ❏ Donnagel
- ❏ Equalactin
- ❏ FiberCon
- ❏ Furoxone
- ❏ furazolidone
- ❏ Homapin
- ❏ Imodium
- ❏ Imodium A-D
- ❏ Kaolin
- ❏ Kaopectate
- ❏ Konsyl
- ❏ Lactinex

| ■ | F |
|---|---|

- ❑ Lomotil
- ❑ loperamide
- ❑ Lotronex
- ❑ lubiprostone
- ❑ Metamucil
- ❑ Milk of Bismuth
- ❑ Motofen
- ❑ Mycifradin
- ❑ nitazoxanide
- ❑ Palsorb
- ❑ Paocin
- ❑ Paragel
- ❑ Paralixer
- ❑ Parepectolin
- ❑ Pectocel
- ❑ Pepto-Bismol
- ❑ rifaximin
- ❑ Rotarix
- ❑ Rotateq
- ❑ rotavirus
- ❑ Xifaxan

## ■ FERTILITY

- ❑ anti-phospholipids
- ❑ A.P.L.
- ❑ apomorphine
- ❑ ArginMax
- ❑ Avimil
- ❑ Bravelle
- ❑ Bromocriptine
- ❑ cabergoline
- ❑ Cervidil
- ❑ Cetrorelix
- ❑ Cetrotide
- ❑ Chorex
- ❑ choriogonadotropin alfa
- ❑ chorionic gonadotropin
- ❑ Choron
- ❑ Cialis
- ❑ Clomid
- ❑ clomiphene citrate

| ■ | F |
|---|---|

- ❑ Corgonject
- ❑ Crinone
- ❑ Delestrogen
- ❑ Dostinex
- ❑ Edex
- ❑ Endometrin
- ❑ Fertinex
- ❑ Follistim
- ❑ Follistim/Antagon Kit
- ❑ follitropin alfa/beta
- ❑ Follutein
- ❑ Glukor
- ❑ Gonadorelin
- ❑ Gonal
- ❑ Gonic
- ❑ Humegon
- ❑ Interex
- ❑ Levitra
- ❑ Livial
- ❑ Lutrepulse
- ❑ menotropin
- ❑ Metrodin
- ❑ Muse
- ❑ Novarel
- ❑ Ovidrel
- ❑ Parlodel
- ❑ Pergonal
- ❑ phentolamine
- ❑ Pregnyl
- ❑ Procylon
- ❑ Profasi
- ❑ progesterone
- ❑ Repronex
- ❑ Serephene
- ❑ tadalafil
- ❑ Tibolone
- ❑ Uprima
- ❑ urofollitropin
- ❑ Vasomax
- ❑ Viagra
- ❑ Yohimex

| G | H |
|---|---|

☐ Yokon

**■ HEMORRHAGE**
☐ adrenalin chloride

**■ GLAUCOMA**
☐ acetazolamide
☐ AkPro
☐ Alphagan
☐ Azopt
☐ betaxolol
☐ Betoptic
☐ brimonidine
☐ brinzolamide
☐ carbachol
☐ Carbastat
☐ Carboptic
☐ Cosopt
☐ Daranide
☐ demecarium
☐ Diamox
☐ Diamox Sequels
☐ dichlorphenamide
☐ dipivefrin
☐ dorzolamide
☐ echothiophate
☐ Epifrin
☐ Epinal
☐ epinephrine
☐ Eppy/N
☐ Eserine
☐ Floropryl
☐ Humorsol
☐ isoflurophate
☐ isopto carbachol
☐ isopto carpine
☐ isopto eserine
☐ latanoprost
☐ Miostat
☐ phospholine iodide
☐ physostigmine
☐ Trusopt
☐ Zalatan

☐ Aggrastat
☐ albumin
☐ AlphaNine SD
☐ Amicar
☐ aminocaproic acid
☐ aprotinin
☐ Arixtra
☐ Autoplex
☐ Avitene
☐ BeneFix
☐ cellulose, oxidized
☐ Cyklokapron
☐ factor IX complex
☐ Flexbumin
☐ gelatin (absorbable)
☐ Gelfilm
☐ Gelfoam
☐ Helistat
☐ Hemofil
☐ Hemonyne
☐ Hemotene
☐ Konyne 80
☐ Methergine
☐ methylergonovine
☐ microfibrillar collagen
☐ Mononine
☐ nimodipine
☐ Nimotop
☐ NovoSeven
☐ Oxycel
☐ Profilnine SD
☐ Proplex
☐ Surgicel
☐ Tesseel VH Fibrin Sealant
☐ Thrombinar
☐ tranexamic acid
☐ thrombin
☐ Thrombogen
☐ Thrombostat

| ■ | M |
|---|---|

- ☐ Tirofiban
- ☐ Trasylol

## ■ MALE DRUGS

- ☐ 5-aminosalicylic acid
- ☐ ABX-EGF
- ☐ alprostadil
- ☐ Andro-Teston
- ☐ Asacol
- ☐ Azo-Gantrisin
- ☐ alfuzosin
- ☐ Avodart
- ☐ Bactrim
- ☐ Baridium
- ☐ biclutamide
- ☐ Buserelin
- ☐ Canasa
- ☐ Cardura
- ☐ Casodex
- ☐ Caspofungin
- ☐ Caverject
- ☐ Cialis
- ☐ Cotrim
- ☐ Degarelix
- ☐ Delatestryl
- ☐ Depo-Provera
- ☐ Doxazosin
- ☐ dutasteride
- ☐ Eligard
- ☐ Enzyte
- ☐ Exisulind
- ☐ finasteride
- ☐ Flomax
- ☐ Floxin
- ☐ fluoxymesterone
- ☐ Fortigel
- ☐ Goserelin
- ☐ Halotestin
- ☐ Hytrin
- ☐ IFEX
- ☐ Ifosamide

- ☐ Interex
- ☐ Intimex
- ☐ leuprolide
- ☐ Levitra
- ☐ Livia
- ☐ LoCholest
- ☐ Lupron
- ☐ Maintain
- ☐ ManDelay
- ☐ mesalamine
- ☐ MUSE
- ☐ Nilandron
- ☐ nilutamide
- ☐ ofloxacin
- ☐ PC SPES
- ☐ PDE5 blocker
- ☐ PDE5 inhibitor
- ☐ Pentasa
- ☐ Phen-Azo
- ☐ phenazopyridine
- ☐ phentolamine
- ☐ phosphodiesterase blocker
- ☐ phosphodiesterase inhibitor
- ☐ phytosterol blocker
- ☐ Prevalite
- ☐ Procylon
- ☐ Proscar
- ☐ prostaglandin El
- ☐ pygeum
- ☐ Questran
- ☐ quinolone
- ☐ Rapaflo
- ☐ Rowasa
- ☐ saw palmetto
- ☐ Septra
- ☐ sildenafil citrate
- ☐ silodosin
- ☐ Striant
- ☐ sulfamethoprim
- ☐ Sulfatrim
- ☐ sulfonamide

| ■ | M |
|---|---|

- ❏ Suprefact
- ❏ tadalafil
- ❏ tamsulosin
- ❏ terazosin
- ❏ teriparatide
- ❏ testosterone enanthate
- ❏ Trelstar Depot
- ❏ Trelstar LA
- ❏ Tribolone
- ❏ triptorelin pamoate
- ❏ Ultra ZN
- ❏ Uprima
- ❏ UroXatral
- ❏ Urodine
- ❏ Urogesic
- ❏ Uroplus
- ❏ Vantas
- ❏ vardenafil
- ❏ Vasclip
- ❏ Vasomax
- ❏ Viadur
- ❏ Viagra
- ❏ Vinarol
- ❏ Viridium
- ❏ Yocon
- ❏ Yohimbine
- ❏ Zoladex

## ■ MEDICAL PRODUCTS

- ❏ AB-AUK 3
- ❏ Abbott HCV EIA 2.0
- ❏ AB-COREK
- ❏ Activa Dystonia
- ❏ AcuTect
- ❏ AdreView
- ❏ Agarose gel
- ❏ Alcon Laser
- ❏ AMBU bag
- ❏ Amicar
- ❏ Amino-cerv
- ❏ AneuVysion Assay

- ❏ Apligraf
- ❏ Ascensia Breeze
- ❏ AUK-3
- ❏ AUSAB
- ❏ Bandages
  - HemCon
  - QuickClot
  - RDH
  - TraumaDex
- ❏ Bekesy audiometry
- ❏ Betadine
- ❏ bethanechol
- ❏ BioZ monitor
- ❏ ChloraPrep
- ❏ Cidex scrub
- ❏ Claris
- ❏ COBAS AmpliScreen
- ❏ Cope's needle
- ❏ Cordran Tape
- ❏ Corzyme
- ❏ Coupler
- ❏ curette
- ❏ Custodiol HTK
- ❏ CV Peri-Gard
- ❏ Cypher stent
- ❏ cystourethroscope
- ❏ Dacriose
- ❏ Dermacil tape
- ❏ Derma-Sorb
- ❏ diatrizoate
- ❏ Doppler probe
- ❏ Doppler stethoscope
- ❏ Dropperettes
- ❏ drug-eluting stent
- ❏ Duoderm
- ❏ ELESR
- ❏ Epitope OraSure
- ❏ ETI-AB-AUK
- ❏ ETI-AB-COREK
- ❏ ETI-MAK 2
- ❏ Evicel

| ■ | M |
|---|---|

- ❑ EZ MedTest
- ❑ fetal heart monitor
- ❑ Fibrin Sealant [Tisseel]
- ❑ Flexstent
- ❑ FloThru
- ❑ Fluorognost HIV-IIFA
- ❑ flurandrenolide
- ❑ forceps
- ❑ Gelfilm
- ❑ Gelfoam
- ❑ GentleWave
- ❑ Germa-Medica
- ❑ Giladel wafer
- ❑ glacial acetic acid
- ❑ Gore-Tex
- ❑ Granulex
- ❑ gurney
- ❑ gum guaiac
- ❑ Gynecare ThermaChoice
- ❑ Harrington rod
- ❑ HemCon
- ❑ hemostat
- ❑ Hep-Lock flush
- ❑ HER2/neu
- ❑ Hex-Germ
- ❑ Hibiclens
- ❑ Hibistat hand rinse
- ❑ Hibistat towelette
- ❑ HIVAB HIV-I EIA
- ❑ HydraSorb
- ❑ hydrocollator
- ❑ lamin
- ❑ Instat collagen
- ❑ Instat MCH
- ❑ Insync Model III
- ❑ iobenguane
- ❑ Kaltostat
- ❑ Lap-Band
- ❑ laryngoscope
- ❑ Lasik eye surgery
- ❑ Luer-Lock syringe

| ■ | M |
|---|---|

- ❑ Luffa boots
- ❑ MAST trousers
- ❑ Menocheck
- ❑ Merci Retreiver
- ❑ methacrylate resin
- ❑ microfibrillar
- ❑ micropipette
- ❑ Miraluma test
- ❑ MUREX SUDS HIV
- ❑ Muro Gonio gel
- ❑ Neuromag
- ❑ NG-tube
- ❑ NucliSense HIV I QT
- ❑ Ocu-Gard
- ❑ On-Q
- ❑ OraQuick
- ❑ Ortho Hbc ELISA
- ❑ Ortho HCV
- ❑ Orthotec Products
- ❑ orthotic
- ❑ orthotolidin
- ❑ OsmoCyte
- ❑ otoscope
- ❑ Panafil
- ❑ Panafil SE
- ❑ Pathiam
- ❑ pentagasgtrin
- ❑ Peri-Gard
- ❑ Peri-Strips
- ❑ pHisoHex
- ❑ PLAS+SD
- ❑ polifeprosan
- ❑ potassium hydroxide
- ❑ povidone-iodine
- ❑ PreScrub
- ❑ Procleix
- ❑ ProClude
- ❑ protamine sulfate
- ❑ Puri-Clens
- ❑ QuickClot
- ❑ RDH Bandage

| ■ | M |
|---|---|

- ☐ Renacidin
- ☐ RESPeRATE
- ☐ Reveal Rapid HIV-1
- ☐ Ringer's lactate
- ☐ rLAV EIA
- ☐ Roche Amplicor
- ☐ rongeur forceps
- ☐ Rotablator
- ☐ Saf-Gel
- ☐ SCS Anterior
- ☐ Sea-Clens
- ☐ Septisol
- ☐ shunt
- ☐ Silimed Products
- ☐ speculum
- ☐ stents
  - Chromoflex
  - Cypher
  - Dinatek
  - drug-eleuting
  - Flexstent
  - Guidant
  - Nitinol
  - Pro-Long
  - S-Flex
- ☐ stockinette
- ☐ supernatant
- ☐ Surgasoap
- ☐ Surgibone
- ☐ Surgical Nu-Knit
- ☐ Surgicel
- ☐ Surgidine
- ☐ Surgi-Kleen
- ☐ Surgilube
- ☐ sutures
  - absorbable
  - Alcon
  - caprosyn
  - Chromic
  - Dacron
  - Deknatel

| ■ | M |
|---|---|

- Dermalon
- Ethicon
- Indermil
- Medrafil
- Mersilene
- Perma-Hand
- polyglycolic
- polysorb
- Prolene
- swaged
- ☐ sutures [continued]
  - Tevdek
  - Ti-Cron
  - Vicryl
- ☐ Synovis Products
- ☐ TAXUS Express 2
- ☐ TENS unit
- ☐ Thermage
- ☐ Tisseel VH Fibrin Sealant
- ☐ thermistors
- ☐ ThinPrep
- ☐ tourniquet
- ☐ TraumaDex Bandage
- ☐ Triad
- ☐ Trugene HIV 1
- ☐ Ultraqual HIV-1 RT-Pcr
- ☐ Urecholine
- ☐ wavefront-guided laser
- ☐ Vasclip
- ☐ Vascu-Gard
- ☐ Versant HIV-1 RNA
- ☐ Vironostika HIV-1
- ☐ ViroSeq HIV-1
- ☐ Visx laser surgery
- ☐ Vivosil
- ☐ Water-Jel
- ☐ Woun'dres

**■ MUSCLE RELAXANTS**

- ☐ Amrix
- ☐ Antiflex

| ■ | M | ■ | M |
|---|---|---|---|

- Ativan
- Atracurium Besylate
- Baclofen
- Banflex
- Blanax
- Carbacot
- carisoprodol
- chlorphenesin
- chlorzoxazone
- curare
- cyclobenzaprine
- Dantrium
- Dantrolene
- Delaxin
- diazepam
- Disipal
- Dizac
- Donnatal
- doxacurium chloride
- Flavoxate HCl
- Flaxedil
- Flexagin
- Flexain
- Flexaphen
- Flexeril
- Flexoject
- Flexon
- gallamine triethiodide
- hexafluorenium
- K-Flex
- Lioresal
- Marbaxin
- Marflex
- mephenesin
- meprobamate
- Mestinon
- metaxalone
- methocarbamol
- metocurine iodide
- Metubine
- Mivacron

- mivacurium chloride
- Myolin
- Myotrol
- Neocyten
- Neostig
- neostigmine
- Nimbex
- Noradex
- Norcuron
- Norflex
- Norgesic
- Nuromax
- O-Flex
- Orflagen
- Orfro
- orphenadrine
- orphanagesic
- Orphanate
- Papavirine
- Paraflex
- Parafon
- P-A-V
- phenobarbital
- prostigmin
- pyridostigmine
- Rela
- Relagesic
- Remular
- Robamol
- Robaxin
- Robaxisal
- Robomol
- rocuronium bromide
- Skelaxin
- Skelex
- Sodol
- Soma Compound
- Sopridol
- Soridol
- succinylcholine
- Tega-Flex

| ■ | N |
|---|---|

- ☐ tizanidine
- ☐ Tracrium
- ☐ Tubocurarine
- ☐ Urispas
- ☐ Valrelease
- ☐ vecuronium bromide
- ☐ Zanaflex
- ☐ Zemuron

## ■ NEUROLOGY

- ☐ acetazolamide
- ☐ Adderall
- ☐ Akineton
- ☐ alglucosidase alfa
- ☐ Amantadine
- ☐ Ambenonium
- ☐ Amerge
- ☐ amobarbital
- ☐ amytal
- ☐ Antegren
- ☐ Apokyn
- ☐ apomorphine hydrochloride
- ☐ Aricept
- ☐ armodafinil
- ☐ Artane
- ☐ Atamet
- ☐ Atretol
- ☐ Avonex
- ☐ Azilect
- ☐ Banzel
- ☐ Benedryl
- ☐ benzetropine mesylate
- ☐ Betaseron
- ☐ Biocadren
- ☐ Biperiden
- ☐ Bromocriptine
- ☐ carbamazepine
- ☐ Carbatrol
- ☐ Carbex
- ☐ carbidopa/levodopa
- ☐ Celontin

| ■ | N |
|---|---|

- ☐ Cerebyx
- ☐ Cevimeline
- ☐ Clindets
- ☐ clonazepam
- ☐ clorazepate
- ☐ Cogentin
- ☐ Cognex
- ☐ Concerta
- ☐ Copaxone
- ☐ Cylert
- ☐ Cymbalta
- ☐ Dantrium
- ☐ Decadron
- ☐ Deltasone
- ☐ Depacon
- ☐ Depakene
- ☐ Depakote
- ☐ Depo-Medrol
- ☐ Desoxyn
- ☐ dexamethasone
- ☐ Dexedrine
- ☐ Dextrostat
- ☐ dextroamphetamine sulfate
- ☐ DHE 45
- ☐ Diamox
- ☐ difluprednate
- ☐ dihydroergotamine
- ☐ Dilantin
- ☐ diphenhydramine
- ☐ Diphenylan
- ☐ divalproex sodium
- ☐ Donepezil
- ☐ Dopram
- ☐ Dornase Alfa
- ☐ duloxetine
- ☐ Durezol
- ☐ edrophonium chloride
- ☐ Eldepryl
- ☐ Epitol
- ☐ Epsol
- ☐ Ergomar

| | N | | | N |
|---|---|---|---|---|

- ❑ ergotamine
- ❑ Estorra
- ❑ eszopiclone
- ❑ ethosuximide
- ❑ Ethotoin
- ❑ Evoxac
- ❑ Exelon
- ❑ Felbamate
- ❑ Felbatol
- ❑ fosphenytoin
- ❑ Gabapentin
- ❑ Gabitril
- ❑ Gamunex
- ❑ Gen-Xene
- ❑ Haldol
- ❑ Halperidol
- ❑ HepaGam B
- ❑ hydroxychloroquine
- ❑ Imitrex
- ❑ Increlex
- ❑ Inderal
- ❑ interferon
- ❑ interferon Beta-1A
- ❑ interferon Beta-1B
- ❑ Invega
- ❑ isoxsuprine
- ❑ Kemadrin
- ❑ Keppra
- ❑ Klonopin
- ❑ lacosamide
- ❑ Lamictal
- ❑ lamotrigine
- ❑ lanreotide acetate
- ❑ Larodopa
- ❑ Levbid
- ❑ levetiracetam
- ❑ Levsin
- ❑ Levsinex
- ❑ Lamictal
- ❑ Lamotrigine
- ❑ lisdexamfetamine dimesylate

- ❑ Lodosyn
- ❑ Luminal
- ❑ Lunesta
- ❑ Lyrica
- ❑ magnesium sulfate
- ❑ Maxalt
- ❑ Mebaral
- ❑ mecasermin
- ❑ Medrol
- ❑ Mephenytoin
- ❑ mephobarbital
- ❑ Mesantoin
- ❑ Mestinon
- ❑ methamphetamine
- ❑ Methsuximide
- ❑ methylphenidate
- ❑ methylprednisolone
- ❑ Midrin
- ❑ midocrine
- ❑ Migranal nasal spray
- ❑ milnacipran
- ❑ Milontin
- ❑ Mirapex
- ❑ Modafinil
- ❑ Myozyme
- ❑ Mysoline
- ❑ Mytelase caplets
- ❑ naratriptan
- ❑ Nascobal
- ❑ natalizumab
- ❑ Neostigmine
- ❑ Neupro
- ❑ Neurontin
- ❑ Novantrone
- ❑ Nuvigil
- ❑ Orap
- ❑ Orapred
- ❑ Orasone
- ❑ oxazepam
- ❑ oxcarbazepine
- ❑ Oxytrol

| ■ | N |
|---|---|

- ❑ paliperidone
- ❑ Parcopa
- ❑ Pemoline
- ❑ Parlodel
- ❑ Pediapred
- ❑ Peganone
- ❑ Pergolide
- ❑ Permax
- ❑ phenobarbital
- ❑ phensuximide
- ❑ Phenytek
- ❑ Phenytoin
- ❑ Pimozide
- ❑ Plaquenil
- ❑ pramipexole
- ❑ prednisolone
- ❑ prednisone
- ❑ pregabalin
- ❑ Prestara
- ❑ Primidone
- ❑ ProAmatine
- ❑ propranolol
- ❑ Prostigmin
- ❑ Provigil
- ❑ Pulmozyme
- ❑ Pyridostigmine
- ❑ ramelteon
- ❑ rasagiline mesylate
- ❑ Rebif
- ❑ Regonol
- ❑ Requip
- ❑ Rilutek
- ❑ Riluzole
- ❑ rivastigmine
- ❑ rizatriptan
- ❑ ropinirole
- ❑ rotigotine
- ❑ Rozerem
- ❑ rufinamide
- ❑ Savella
- ❑ Selegiline

| ■ | N |
|---|---|

- ❑ Sinemet
- ❑ Sodium Oxybate
- ❑ Solu-Medrol
- ❑ Somatuline Autogel
- ❑ Somatuline Depot
- ❑ Stalevo
- ❑ Stavzor
- ❑ succinimide
- ❑ sumatriptan
- ❑ Symmetrel
- ❑ Tacrine
- ❑ Tasmar
- ❑ Tegretol
- ❑ Tensilon
- ❑ Tercica
- ❑ tetrabenazine
- ❑ tiagabine
- ❑ timolol maleate
- ❑ tizanidine
- ❑ TOBI
- ❑ Tobramycin
- ❑ Tolcapone
- ❑ Topamax
- ❑ topiramate
- ❑ Tranxene
- ❑ Tridione
- ❑ trihexyphenidyl
- ❑ Trileptal
- ❑ trimethadione
- ❑ TVP-1012
- ❑ Tysabri
- ❑ Valium
- ❑ valproic acid
- ❑ Vimpat
- ❑ Vyvanse
- ❑ Wigraine
- ❑ Xenazine
- ❑ Xyrem
- ❑ Zanalfex
- ❑ Zarontin
- ❑ Zelapar

| ■ | ○ | | ■ | ○ |

- ❑ Zolmitriptan
- ❑ Zolpidem
- ❑ Zolpimist
- ❑ Zomig
- ❑ Zonegran
- ❑ zonisamide

## ■ OBESITY

- ❑ Acomplia
- ❑ Adipex
- ❑ Adipex-P
- ❑ Adipost
- ❑ Adphen
- ❑ AdvantEdge
- ❑ Alli
- ❑ Anorex
- ❑ Anoxine
- ❑ Appecon
- ❑ Aqua-Ban
- ❑ Axokine
- ❑ AYDS
- ❑ benzphetamine
- ❑ BioLean
- ❑ BioMD Nutraceuticals
- ❑ Biotest Hot-Rox
- ❑ Bontril PDM
- ❑ Carb Cutter
- ❑ Chroma Slim
- ❑ Dapex
- ❑ desoxyn
- ❑ Dexatrim
- ❑ dexfenfluramine
- ❑ Didrex
- ❑ diethylpropion
- ❑ Dital
- ❑ Dyrexan
- ❑ EAS Thermo DynamX
- ❑ Estrin-D
- ❑ Exgest LA
- ❑ fenfluramine
- ❑ Fen-Phen

- ❑ Hydroxycut
- ❑ Ionamin
- ❑ Isatori Lean
- ❑ Leptoprin
- ❑ LipoTrim
- ❑ Mazindol
- ❑ Mazinor
- ❑ Medifast
- ❑ Meridia
- ❑ Metab-O-Fx
- ❑ Metabolife
- ❑ methamphetamine
- ❑ MHP TakeOff Hi-Energy
- ❑ M-Orexic
- ❑ Natrol
- ❑ Natrol CitriMax
- ❑ Nature's Bounty Xtreme Lean
- ❑ Nunaturals LevelRight
- ❑ Obalan
- ❑ Obenix
- ❑ Obe-Del
- ❑ Obe-Mar
- ❑ Obe-Nix
- ❑ Obephen
- ❑ Obermine
- ❑ Obestin
- ❑ Obezine
- ❑ Oby-Cap
- ❑ Oby-Trim
- ❑ One-A-Day Weight Smart
- ❑ Orlistat
- ❑ Panrexin
- ❑ Panshape
- ❑ Parzine
- ❑ PatentLean
- ❑ Phendiet
- ❑ phendimetrazine
- ❑ Phentercot
- ❑ phentermine
- ❑ Phentra
- ❑ Phentride

- Phentrol
- phenylpropanolamine
- Phenzine
- Plegine
- Pondimin
- Prelu-2
- Preludin-Endurete
- Prolab
- PT-105
- PureTrim
- Redux
- Rexigen
- rimonabant
- Sanorex
- sibutramine
- Slynn-LL
- Stacker 2
- Statobex
- T-Diet
- Tega-Nil
- Tenuate
- Tenuate Dospan
- Tepanil
- Teramin
- Tetrazene ES-50
- Thermogenics
- Thinz
- ThyroStart
- Trimstat
- Twinlab GTB Chromium
- Wehles
- Wehles Timecelles
- Weightrol
- Xenadrine
- Xenical
- XtremeLean
- X-Trozine LA
- Zantrex
- Zantryl

## ■ OB/GYN

- 17-beta estradiol
- acid jelly
- Aci-Jel
- Aclasta
- Activella
- Activelle
- Actonel
- acyclovir
- adalimumab
- Adipex
- Adipex-P
- Aldara
- alendronate
- Alesse
- Alluna
- Alora
- Amen
- Amerge
- amphotericin
- Amino-Cerv
- anastrozole
- Ancobon
- Angeliq
- anidulafungin
- A.P.L.
- Apri
- ArginMax
- Arimidex
- AVC Cream
- Aviane
- Avlimil
- Aygestin
- Azactim
- AZO
- Bactrim
- Betadine
- Bijuva
- Bio-E-Gel
- Boniva
- Brevicon

- bromocriptine
- BufferGel
- butoconazole
- Cacit
- calcitonin
- Calcitonin-Salmon
- Cancidas
- Canesten
- carboprost
- Carlesta
- caspofungin
- Cellasene
- Cenestin
- Ceptaz
- Cervidil
- Cetrorelix
- Cetrotide
- cholecalciferol
- chorionic gonadotropin
- Cipro
- ciprofloxacin
- CitraNatal
- Clearblue
- Cleocin
- Climara
- Climara Pro
- Clindesse
- Clomid
- clomiphene citrate
- Clotrimaderm
- clotrimazole
- CombiPatch
- Conceptrol
- Condylox
- Crinone
- Cyclen
- Cyclessa
- Cycrin
- Cryselle
- Cystex
- Cystospas

- DawnMist
- DDAVP
- Delestrogen
- Delfen
- Demulin
- Depo-Provera
- depo-subQ provera
- Desmopressin
- Desogen
- desogestrel
- desvenlafaxine
- Detrol
- Detrol LA
- D.H.E.
- dienestrol
- diflucan
- dihydroergotamine
- dinoprostone
- Divigel
- Dong Quai
- drospirenone
- Duralutin
- Duricef
- EC-Naprosyn
- econazole
- Ecostatin
- Edex
- eflornithine
- Elestrin
- Ellence
- EMKO
- Enjuvia
- Enovid
- Enpresse
- Epirubicin
- Eraxis
- Ergomar
- ergotamine tartrate
- Esclim Patch
- Estinyl
- Estrace

- ☐ Estraderm
- ☐ estradiol
- ☐ Estrasorb
- ☐ Estratab
- ☐ Estratest
- ☐ Estratest H.S.
- ☐ Estring
- ☐ EstroGel
- ☐ estrogen
- ☐ estropipate
- ☐ Estrostep
- ☐ ethyl estradiol
- ☐ ethynodiol diacetate
- ☐ Euthoid
- ☐ EvaMist
- ☐ Evista
- ☐ Extrasorb
- ☐ famciclovir
- ☐ Famvir
- ☐ Fareston
- ☐ Faslodex
- ☐ FDS feminine spray
- ☐ Femara
- ☐ Fem-Cap
- ☐ FemCare
- ☐ Femcet
- ☐ Femhrt
- ☐ Femizol
- ☐ Fempatch
- ☐ Femring
- ☐ Femstat
- ☐ Femtrace
- ☐ Fertinex
- ☐ flucytosine
- ☐ fluoxetine
- ☐ Follistim
- ☐ follitropin alfa/beta
- ☐ Fortaz
- ☐ Forteo
- ☐ Fortical
- ☐ Fosamax

- ☐ Fosteum
- ☐ fulvestrant
- ☐ Fungizone
- ☐ Furadantin
- ☐ Gardasil
- ☐ Genapax
- ☐ GenCept
- ☐ genistein aglycone
- ☐ gentian violet
- ☐ Gesterol
- ☐ Gonal
- ☐ Genora
- ☐ Gynazole
- ☐ GyneCure
- ☐ Gyne-Lotrimin
- ☐ Gynix
- ☐ Gynodiol
- ☐ Gyno-Trosyd
- ☐ Hemabate
- ☐ Herceptin
- ☐ Humegon
- ☐ Humira
- ☐ Hy/Gestrone
- ☐ Hylutin
- ☐ HypRho
- ☐ Hyprogest
- ☐ Hyproval P.A.
- ☐ Hyskon
- ☐ ibandronate
- ☐ imiquimod
- ☐ Imitrex
- ☐ Indocin
- ☐ indomethacin
- ☐ Innofem
- ☐ Inti-Mist
- ☐ Intrinsa
- ☐ itraconazole
- ☐ ixabepilone
- ☐ Ixempra
- ☐ Jadelle
- ☐ Jenest

- ☐ Junel
- ☐ Kariva
- ☐ ketoconazole
- ☐ Koo Sar
- ☐ Koromex
- ☐ lanreotide acetate
- ☐ lapatinib
- ☐ Legatrin PM
- ☐ Lessina
- ☐ letrozole
- ☐ Levaquin
- ☐ Levlen
- ☐ Levlite
- ☐ Levora
- ☐ levonorgestrel
- ☐ Levothroid
- ☐ levothyroxine
- ☐ Levoxyl
- ☐ Liotrix
- ☐ Lippes Loop
- ☐ Loestrin
- ☐ Lo/Ovral
- ☐ Low-Ogestrel
- ☐ Lubriderm
- ☐ Lunelle
- ☐ Lupron
- ☐ Lutera
- ☐ lutropin alfa
- ☐ Luveris
- ☐ Lybrel
- ☐ Macrobid
- ☐ Macrodantin
- ☐ Marvelon
- ☐ Massengil products
- ☐ Maxalt
- ☐ Maxipime
- ☐ medroxyprogesterone
- ☐ Megace
- ☐ Menest
- ☐ Menocheck
- ☐ Menostar

- ☐ mentropin
- ☐ Mestranol
- ☐ Methergine
- ☐ metazoline
- ☐ Metrodin
- ☐ MetroGel
- ☐ metronidazole
- ☐ Miacalcin
- ☐ miconazole
- ☐ MICRhoGam
- ☐ Micronor
- ☐ Midol
- ☐ Mifeprex
- ☐ mifepristone
- ☐ MigraHealth
- ☐ Migranal
- ☐ Minestrin
- ☐ Minoxidil
- ☐ Min-Ovral
- ☐ Mircette
- ☐ Mirena
- ☐ ModiCon
- ☐ Monistat
- ☐ Mono-Stat
- ☐ Monuril
- ☐ MUSE
- ☐ Mycelex
- ☐ Myclo
- ☐ Myclo-Gyne
- ☐ Mycostatin
- ☐ M-Zole 3
- ☐ Nadostine
- ☐ Nafarelin
- ☐ naladixic acid
- ☐ naratriptan
- ☐ Necon
- ☐ N.E.E.
- ☐ NegGram
- ☐ Nelova
- ☐ Nelulen
- ☐ Neutrogena products

■ ○ ■ ○

- Nicomide
- nicotinamide
- Nicosyn
- Nilstat
- Nizoral A-D
- Nolvadex
- nonoxynol
- Norcept
- Nordette
- norelgestromin
- norethindrone
- Norgestrel
- Norinyl
- Norlutate
- Norlutin
- Noroxin
- Norplant
- Nor-QD
- Nortrel
- Novo-Miconazole
- Noxafil
- NuvaRing
- Nyaderm
- Nystatin
- Ogen cream
- Ogestrel
- Ortho-Cept
- Ortho-Creme
- Ortho-Cyclen
- Ortho Dienestrol
- Ortho-Est
- Ortho Evra Patch
- Ortho-Gynol
- Ortho-Micronor
- Ortho-Novum
- Ortho-Prefest
- Ortho Tri-Cyclen
- Ortho Tri-Cyclen Lo
- Osteo Bi-Flex
- Ovcon
- Ovidrel

- Ovral
- OvaRex
- Ovrette
- oxytocin
- Oxytrol
- Pamprin
- papillomavirus
- ParaGard T380a
- Parlodel
- Pediapred
- Pediarix
- Penlac polish
- Pergonal
- phytoestrogen
- piperazine estrone
- Pitocin
- Pitressin
- Plan B
- podofilux gel
- Portia
- posaconazole
- prednisolone
- prednisone
- Pregnyl
- Premarin
- Premphase
- Prempro
- Premsyn
- Prepidil
- Prestara
- Primaxin
- Pristiq
- Prochieve
- Pro-Depo
- Progestaject
- progesterone
- progesterone gel
- Progestilin
- Proloid
- Prometrium
- Prosed

- prostaglandine
- Prostin E2
- Provera
- Psorcon
- Pyridium
- quadrivalent
- Radiance injection
- Raloxifene
- Reclast
- Replens
- Repronex
- RespiGam
- risedronate
- ritodrine
- rizatriptan
- Rovamycine
- RU-486
- Sarafem
- SCE-A
- Sedapap
- Semicid
- Septra
- Soltamox
- Somatuline
- Spiramycin
- Sporanox
- Sultran
- sumatriptan
- Symphasic
- Synarel
- Synthroid
- Syntocinon
- tamoxifen
- Terazol
- teriparatide
- testolactone
- ThermaCare
- Tindamax
- tinidazole
- tioconazole
- Tolterodine

- toremifene
- Tri-Levlen
- Tri-Norinyl
- Triphasil
- Tri-Sprintec
- Trivora
- Tropsium
- Tykerb
- Urised
- Urobiotic
- urofollitropin
- Uroquid
- Vagifem
- Vagisil
- Vagistat
- valacyclovir
- Valtrex
- Vaniqa
- Vasopressin
- Venastat
- Viactiv
- Viagra
- Vivelle-Dot
- Wigraine
- WinRho SDF
- Yokon
- Yutopar
- Zaroxolyn
- zoledronic acid
- zolmitriptan
- Zomig
- Zovia
- Zovirax

## ■ OPHTHALMICS
- acetazolamide
- acetylcholine
- Acular
- Adsorbocarpine
- Akarpine
- AK-Con

| ■ | ○ | ■ | ○ |
|---|---|---|---|

- AK-Dilate
- AK-Fluor
- AK-Nefrin
- AK-Pentolate
- AK-Poly-Bac
- AK-Pred
- AK-Spore
- Akten
- Aktob
- AK-Tracin
- AK-Trol
- Akwa Tears
- Alaway
- Alcaine
- Alcon Laser
- Allergan Lacri-Lube
- Almocarpine
- Alomide
- alpha chymar
- alpha chymotrypsin
- alpha lipoic
- Alrex
- Anacel
- AneuVysion Assay
- Antibiopto
- Aosoft
- apraclonidine
- Atropine
- AzaSite
- azithromycin
- Azopt
- bacitracin
- Benoxinate
- benzalkonium
- Betaxon
- Betoptic
- bimatoprost
- Bion Tears
- Bleph-10
- Blephamide
- Blinx

- Botox
- brimonidine tartrate
- brinzolamide
- BSS
- Bufopto
- Carbacel
- Carbachol
- Caterase
- Cetapred
- Chibroxin
- chloramphenicol
- Ciloxan
- Clerz
- Chloromycetin
- Choloroptic
- chymotrypsin
- Collyrium
- Coly-Mycin
- Combigan
- Cortisporin
- cromolyn sodium
- Cromoptic
- Cyclogyl
- cyclopentolate
- cycloplegic
- Dacriose
- dapiprazole
- Daranide
- Definity
- Degest
- demacarium
- dexamethasone
- Diamox
- dichlorphenamide
- difluprednate
- Dilatair
- Dionephrine
- Dorsolamide
- diquafosol tetrasodium
- DuoVisc
- Duratears

- Durezol
- E-Carpine
- Ecodide
- Econochlor
- Econopred
- Efricel
- Elestat
- Emedastine
- Emidine
- Enuclene
- E-Pilo
- Epinal
- epinastine hydrochloride
- erythromycin ethylsuccinate
- ethoxzolamide
- Eyesine
- Fluoracaine
- fluorescein
- fluorometholone
- Fluoroseptic
- Fluress
- FML
- Fomivirsen
- Ful-Glo
- Funduscein
- Ganciclovir
- Gentak
- gentamicin
- GenTeal
- Glaucon
- glutathione
- Herplex
- HMS Liquifilm
- Homatrocel
- Humorsol
- hyaluronidase
- hydroxypropyl
- Hy-Flo
- Hylenex
- Hypersal
- hypromellose

- IC-Green
- Iopidine
- idoxuridine
- Ilotycin
- indocyanine green
- Inflamase
- INS365
- I-Phrine
- Iquix
- Irigate
- Isopto atropine
- Isopto carbachol
- Isopto cetamide
- Isopto eserine
- Istalol
- Ketorolac
- ketotifen
- Lacri-Lube
- Lacrisert
- Lasik eye surgery
- Latisse
- levobetaxolol
- levobunolol
- levofloxacin
- Lopidine
- Lotemax
- Loteprednol
- lodoxamide
- Lucentis
- Lumigan
- Lytears
- Macugen
- Medimyd
- medrysone
- Methopto
- Methulose
- methylcellulose
- Metreton
- Miocarpine
- Miochol
- Mi-Pilo

| ■ | ○ | ■ | ○ |
|---|---|---|---|

- ❑ Murine
- ❑ Murocoll
- ❑ Muro Gonio-Gel
- ❑ Muro ointment
- ❑ Mydriacyl
- ❑ Mydrin
- ❑ Mytrate
- ❑ naphazoline
- ❑ Naphcon A
- ❑ Navstel
- ❑ NeoDecadron
- ❑ Neo-Flo
- ❑ Neo-Frin
- ❑ Neomycin
- ❑ Neo-Synephrine
- ❑ Neozin
- ❑ nepafenac
- ❑ Nevanac
- ❑ Ocu-Carpine
- ❑ Ocuflox
- ❑ OcuFresh
- ❑ Ocugestrin
- ❑ OcuHist
- ❑ Ocu-Mycin
- ❑ Ocu-Phrin
- ❑ Ocusert Pilo
- ❑ Ocusol
- ❑ olopatadine
- ❑ Opcon-A
- ❑ Ophthaine
- ❑ Ophthetic
- ❑ Ophthochlor
- ❑ Ophthocort
- ❑ Opticrom
- ❑ OptiGold
- ❑ Optimyd
- ❑ Optipranolol
- ❑ Optised
- ❑ Optivar
- ❑ papain
- ❑ Pataday

- ❑ Patanol
- ❑ pegaptanib
- ❑ Pemirolast
- ❑ Pereflutren Lipid
- ❑ Phenoptic
- ❑ phenylephrine
- ❑ pheniramine maleate
- ❑ Phospholine
- ❑ Pilocar
- ❑ Pilocarpine
- ❑ Pilocel
- ❑ Pilopine
- ❑ Piloptic
- ❑ Pilostat
- ❑ Polytrim
- ❑ prednisolone
- ❑ prednisone
- ❑ Predulose
- ❑ Prefrin
- ❑ Proparacaine
- ❑ propylene glycol
- ❑ P.V. Carpine
- ❑ Quixin
- ❑ ranibizumab
- ❑ Restasis
- ❑ Retisert
- ❑ Rev-Eyes
- ❑ Rohto Zi
- ❑ Rose Bengal
- ❑ Salagen
- ❑ silver nitrate
- ❑ Spersaphrine
- ❑ Stoxil
- ❑ Sulfacel
- ❑ sulfacetamide
- ❑ Systane
- ❑ Tearisol
- ❑ Tears Naturale
- ❑ Tetracaine
- ❑ tetracycline
- ❑ tetrahydrozoline

## O

- TheraTears
- timolol
- Timoptic in ocudose
- Timoptic-XE
- Travatan Z
- travoprost
- triamcinolone
- tricarbocyanine
- Triesence
- trifluorothymidine
- Trivaris
- tropicamide
- Trusopt
- tyloxapol
- Vasocidin
- Vasocon
- Vasosulf
- verteporfin
- vidarabine
- Vira-A
- Virasert
- Viroptic
- Visine
- Visine-A
- Visine L.R.
- Visx Laser
- Visculose
- Visudyne
- VISUtein
- Vitravene
- Viva-Drops
- wavefront-guided laser
- Xibrom
- Zaditor
- zeaxanthin
- zinc bacitracin
- zinc sulfate
- Zincfren
- Zolyse
- Zylet

## P

### ■ PSYCHOTROPICS

- Abilify
- Abilify Discmelt
- alprazolam
- Ambien
- amitriptyline
- amoxapine
- amphetamine
- Anafranil
- Aplenzin
- aripiprazole
- Asendin
- Atarax
- Ativan
- atomoxetine
- barbiturate
- Benzedrine
- benzodiazepine
- bromazepam
- bupropion
- Buspar
- buspirone
- butabarbital
- Butisol
- carbamazepine
- Campral
- Celexa
- Centrax
- Chantix
- chloral hydrate
- chlordiazepoxide
- chlorpromazine
- Citalopram
- Clindex
- Clinoxide
- clomipramine
- clonazepam
- clorazepate
- clozapine
- Clozaril
- Compazine

| ■ | P | | ■ | P |
|---|---|---|---|---|

- ☐ Concerta
- ☐ Cylert
- ☐ Cymbalta
- ☐ Dalmane
- ☐ Daytrana
- ☐ Depakote
- ☐ desipramine
- ☐ Desoxyn
- ☐ desvenlafaxine
- ☐ Desyrel
- ☐ Dexedrine
- ☐ dexmethylphenidate
- ☐ Diastat
- ☐ diazepam
- ☐ Doral
- ☐ doxepin
- ☐ Droperidol
- ☐ duloxetine
- ☐ Effexor
- ☐ Elavil
- ☐ Emsam
- ☐ Endep
- ☐ Equetro
- ☐ Escitalopram
- ☐ Eskalith
- ☐ estazolam
- ☐ Estorra
- ☐ ethchlorvynol
- ☐ Etrafon
- ☐ FazaClo
- ☐ flunitrazepam
- ☐ fluvoxamine
- ☐ fluoxetine
- ☐ Focalin XR
- ☐ Geodon
- ☐ halazepam
- ☐ Halcion
- ☐ Haldol
- ☐ haloperidol
- ☐ hydrochlorothiazide
- ☐ hydroxyzine pamoate

- ☐ imipramine
- ☐ Indiplon
- ☐ Invega
- ☐ ketazolam
- ☐ Klonopin
- ☐ Lexapro
- ☐ Librax
- ☐ Librium
- ☐ Libritabs
- ☐ Lidoxide
- ☐ Limbitrol
- ☐ lisdexamfetamine dimesylate
- ☐ Lopoxide
- ☐ Lithium
- ☐ Lithobid
- ☐ lorazepam
- ☐ loxapine
- ☐ Loxitane
- ☐ LSD
- ☐ Ludiomil
- ☐ Lunesta
- ☐ Luvox
- ☐ maprotiline
- ☐ Mebaral
- ☐ Medillium
- ☐ Megace
- ☐ megestrol
- ☐ Mellaril
- ☐ mephobarbital
- ☐ meprobamate
- ☐ mesoridazine
- ☐ methylphenidate
- ☐ Meval
- ☐ midazolam
- ☐ Miltown
- ☐ mirtazapine
- ☐ Moban
- ☐ modafinil
- ☐ molindone
- ☐ MTS
- ☐ nafazodone

|  | P |
|---|---|

- ❏ Nardil
- ❏ Navane
- ❏ Nembutal
- ❏ Niravam
- ❏ nitrazepam
- ❏ Norpramin
- ❏ nortriptyline
- ❏ Nu-Alpraz
- ❏ Nu-Loraz
- ❏ olanzapine
- ❏ Oretic
- ❏ Orap
- ❏ oxazepam
- ❏ paliperidone
- ❏ Pamelor
- ❏ Parnate
- ❏ paroxetine
- ❏ Paxil
- ❏ Paxil CR
- ❏ Paxipam
- ❏ pentobarbital
- ❏ perphenazine
- ❏ phencyclidine
- ❏ phenelzine
- ❏ phenothiazide
- ❏ Placidyl
- ❏ PMB 200
- ❏ PMS
- ❏ prazepam
- ❏ Pristiq
- ❏ prochlorperazine
- ❏ Prolixin
- ❏ ProSom
- ❏ protriptyline
- ❏ provigil
- ❏ Prozac
- ❏ Quaalude
- ❏ quazepam
- ❏ quetiapine
- ❏ ramelteon
- ❏ Remeron

- ❏ REMERONSolTab
- ❏ Restoril
- ❏ Risperdal
- ❏ risperidone
- ❏ Ritalin
- ❏ Rivotril
- ❏ Rohypnol
- ❏ Roofie
- ❏ Rozerem
- ❏ Sarafem
- ❏ Seconal
- ❏ selegiline
- ❏ Sepracor
- ❏ Serax
- ❏ Serentil
- ❏ Seroquel
- ❏ sertraline
- ❏ Serzone
- ❏ Sinequan
- ❏ sodium brevital
- ❏ sodium pentothal
- ❏ sodium seconal
- ❏ Solium
- ❏ Somnol
- ❏ Sonata
- ❏ Stavzor
- ❏ Stelazine
- ❏ Strattera
- ❏ Surmontil
- ❏ Symbyax
- ❏ temazepam
- ❏ thiothixine
- ❏ thiordazine
- ❏ Thorazine
- ❏ Tofranil
- ❏ T-Quil
- ❏ Trancopal
- ❏ tranylcypromine sulfate
- ❏ Tranxene
- ❏ trazodone
- ❏ Triavil

## S

- ☐ triazolam
- ☐ Trilafon
- ☐ trimipramine maleate
- ☐ Valium
- ☐ valproic
- ☐ Valrelease
- ☐ varenicline
- ☐ venlafaxine
- ☐ Vistaril
- ☐ Vivactil
- ☐ Vivol
- ☐ Vyvanse
- ☐ Wellbutrin
- ☐ Xanax
- ☐ Zaleplon
- ☐ Zapex
- ☐ Zetran
- ☐ ziprasidone
- ☐ Zoloft
- ☐ Zolpidem Tartrate
- ☐ Zolpimist
- ☐ Zyprexa

## ■ SHOCK

- ☐ albumin
- ☐ aminocaproic acid
- ☐ Dalalone
- ☐ Decadron
- ☐ Decaject
- ☐ dexamethasone
- ☐ Dexasone
- ☐ Dexone
- ☐ Dextran
- ☐ dextrose in NaCl
- ☐ dextrose in water
- ☐ dopamine
- ☐ Flexbumin
- ☐ Gentran
- ☐ Hexadrol
- ☐ hydrocortisone
- ☐ Intropin

## U

- ☐ isoproterenol
- ☐ Macrodex
- ☐ methylprednisolone
- ☐ Neo-Synephrine
- ☐ phenylephrine
- ☐ Plasmanate
- ☐ Plasma-Plex
- ☐ plasma protein fraction
- ☐ Plasmatein
- ☐ Protenate
- ☐ Rheomacrodex
- ☐ Solurex

## ■ UROLOGY

- ☐ Aci-Jel
- ☐ Aldara
- ☐ aldesleukin
- ☐ allopurinol
- ☐ amino acid injection
- ☐ Aminosyn
- ☐ Amoxil
- ☐ Amphotec
- ☐ amphotericin
- ☐ ampicillin
- ☐ Ancobon
- ☐ Androderm
- ☐ Android
- ☐ Andro-L.A.
- ☐ Andropository
- ☐ Atrosept
- ☐ Augmentin
- ☐ Azactam
- ☐ aztreonam
- ☐ Bactrim
- ☐ bethanechol
- ☐ Bethaprim
- ☐ BranchAmin
- ☐ bumetanide
- ☐ Calcibind
- ☐ Capen
- ☐ Captimer

| U | U |
|---|---|

- Cardura
- Ceclor
- cefepime
- cefixime
- cefmetazole
- Cefobid
- cefonicid
- cefoperazone
- Ceftin
- ceftizoxime
- cefuroxime
- Ceptaz
- cholesteryl
- Cinobac
- cinoxacin
- Cipro
- ciprofloxacin
- Claforan
- Clorpactin
- clotrimazole
- Condylox
- conivaptan
- Cotrim
- Cuprimine
- Cymbalta
- Cystagon
- cysteamine
- Cystospaz
- darifenacin
- DDAVP
- Delatest
- Delatestryl
- depAndro
- Depen
- Depotest
- Depo Testosterone
- desmopressin
- Detrol
- Detrol LA
- dimethyl sulfoxide
- Ditropan

- Ditropan XL
- Dolsed
- Doribax
- doripenem
- Doryx
- doxercalciferol
- duloxetine
- Duratest
- Durathate
- Duricef
- Duvoid
- Elmiron
- Enablex
- Epatiol
- Everone
- Ethyol
- fesoterodine fumarate
- Flomax
- Flovoxate
- Fortaz
- fosfomycin
- Fosrenol
- FreAmine
- Fungizone
- Furadantin
- Furalan
- Furan
- Furanite
- gatifloxacin
- Hectorol
- HepatAmine
- Hipex
- Histerone
- hyaluronidase
- Hylenex
- hyoscyamine
- Hytrin
- imipenem
- imiquimod
- Keflex
- ketoconazole

| ■ | U | ■ | U |
|---|---|---|---|

- [ ] K-Phos
- [ ] lanthanum carbonate
- [ ] Levaquin
- [ ] Lithostat
- [ ] leuprolide
- [ ] Levaquin
- [ ] levofloxacin
- [ ] Lorabid
- [ ] Loracarbef
- [ ] Lotrim
- [ ] Lupron
- [ ] Lyphocin
- [ ] Macrobid
- [ ] Macrodantin
- [ ] Mandelamine
- [ ] Mannitol
- [ ] Maxipime
- [ ] Mesna
- [ ] MESNIX
- [ ] methenamine
- [ ] methyltestosterone
- [ ] mezlocillin
- [ ] Monodox
- [ ] Monurol
- [ ] Mucolysin
- [ ] Mycelex
- [ ] nalidixic acid
- [ ] NegGram
- [ ] Neomycin
- [ ] Neosporin
- [ ] NephrAmine
- [ ] nitrofurantoin
- [ ] Nizoral A-D
- [ ] norfloxacin
- [ ] Noroxin
- [ ] Novamine
- [ ] NuLev
- [ ] ofloxacin
- [ ] Oreton Methyl
- [ ] oxybutynin
- [ ] oxytetracycline

- [ ] penicillamine
- [ ] pentosan polysulfate
- [ ] piperacillin
- [ ] Podocon
- [ ] podofilox
- [ ] potassium citrate
- [ ] Polycitra
- [ ] Primaxin
- [ ] Primsol
- [ ] ProcalAmine
- [ ] Prodium
- [ ] Proloprim
- [ ] Proquin XR
- [ ] Proscar
- [ ] Prosed
- [ ] Protrin
- [ ] Pyridium
- [ ] Renacidin
- [ ] Renagel
- [ ] RenAmin
- [ ] Rimso
- [ ] Rocephin
- [ ] Sanctura
- [ ] Sanctura XR
- [ ] Sensipar
- [ ] Septra
- [ ] solifenacin succinate
- [ ] sulfamethoprim
- [ ] Sulfaprim
- [ ] sulfathiazole
- [ ] Sulfoxaprim
- [ ] Sultrin
- [ ] Sutilan
- [ ] Tequin
- [ ] Terazol
- [ ] terconazole
- [ ] Tesamone
- [ ] Testoderm
- [ ] Testopel Pellet
- [ ] Thiola
- [ ] ticarcillin & clavulanate

| ■ | V |
|---|---|

- ☐ Timentin
- ☐ Tioglis
- ☐ tiopronin
- ☐ tolterodine
- ☐ torsemide
- ☐ Toviaz
- ☐ Travasol
- ☐ trimethoprim
- ☐ Trimpex
- ☐ TrophAmine
- ☐ trospium
- ☐ trospium chloride
- ☐ Urecholine
- ☐ Urex
- ☐ Uricalm
- ☐ Urimax
- ☐ Urised
- ☐ Urispas
- ☐ Uritin
- ☐ UroXatral
- ☐ Urobiotic
- ☐ Urocit
- ☐ Uroquid
- ☐ Uroplus
- ☐ Vagistat
- ☐ Vancocin
- ☐ Vantin
- ☐ Vaprisol
- ☐ Vesicare
- ☐ Vibramycin
- ☐ Vibra-Tabs
- ☐ Vinarol
- ☐ Vincol
- ☐ Virilon
- ☐ Vivelle
- ☐ Zinacef
- ☐ Zithromax
- ☐ Zyloprim

## ■ VACCINES

- ☐ H5NI

| ■ | V |
|---|---|

- ☐ ACAM2000
- ☐ Acel-Imune
- ☐ ActHIB
- ☐ Adacel
- ☐ Advate
- ☐ Afluria
- ☐ Aidsvax
- ☐ Anthrax
- ☐ Attenuvax
- ☐ Bacillus Calmette-Guerin
- ☐ Bay-Gam
- ☐ Bay-Hep
- ☐ Bay-Rab
- ☐ Bay-Rho
- ☐ Bay-Tet
- ☐ BIAVAX
- ☐ BioThrax
- ☐ Boostrix
- ☐ Calmette-Guerin
- ☐ Certiva
- ☐ Cholera
- ☐ Comvax
- ☐ CytoGam
- ☐ Daptacel
- ☐ Digibind
- ☐ diphtheria
- ☐ DTP
- ☐ Dryvax
- ☐ Engerix-B
- ☐ Fluarix
- ☐ FluLaval
- ☐ Fluogen
- ☐ FluShield
- ☐ Fluvirin
- ☐ Fluzone
- ☐ Gamimune
- ☐ Gammagard
- ☐ Gammar
- ☐ Gardasil
- ☐ Haemophilus B
- ☐ Havrix

| ■ | V |
|---|---|

- ☐ H-Big
- ☐ HDCV
- ☐ hepatitis
- ☐ Hibtiter
- ☐ HyperRab
- ☐ HyperTet
- ☐ HypRho-D
- ☐ Imogam
- ☐ Imovax
- ☐ Infanrix
- ☐ influenza
- ☐ IPOL
- ☐ IPV
- ☐ Iveegam
- ☐ Je-Vax
- ☐ Kinrix
- ☐ LYMErix
- ☐ Measles
- ☐ Menactra
- ☐ Menomune
- ☐ Meruvax
- ☐ MicrhoGam
- ☐ Movax
- ☐ M-M-R
- ☐ M-R Vax
- ☐ Mumpsvax
- ☐ Nab-HB
- ☐ OKA
- ☐ OmniHIB
- ☐ Optaflu
- ☐ OPV
- ☐ Orimune
- ☐ OspA
- ☐ PedvaxHIB
- ☐ Pentacel
- ☐ Pertusis
- ☐ Pneumovax
- ☐ Pnu-Immune
- ☐ poliomyelitis
- ☐ Poliovax
- ☐ Prevnar

| ■ | V |
|---|---|

- ☐ ProHIBiT
- ☐ Proquad
- ☐ RabAvert
- ☐ Recombinant QspA
- ☐ Recombivax HB
- ☐ RhoGAM
- ☐ Rickettsia
- ☐ Rotarix
- ☐ RotaShield
- ☐ rotavirus
- ☐ Rubella
- ☐ Rubeola
- ☐ Sabin
- ☐ Salk
- ☐ Sandoglobulin
- ☐ smallpox
- ☐ T.A.B.
- ☐ Takeda pertussis
- ☐ TE Anatoxal Berna
- ☐ Tetanus toxoid
- ☐ Tetramune
- ☐ Theracys
- ☐ TICE BCG
- ☐ TOPV
- ☐ TriHibit
- ☐ Tri-Immunol
- ☐ Tripedia
- ☐ tuberculosis
- ☐ Twinrix
- ☐ Typhim
- ☐ Typhoid
- ☐ vaccinia
- ☐ Vaqta
- ☐ varicella
- ☐ Varivax
- ☐ Vivotef Berna
- ☐ VZIG
- ☐ WinRho
- ☐ whooping cough
- ☐ YF-Vax
- ☐ Zemaira

| ■ | X |
|---|---|

- ❏ Zostavax
- **■ X-RAY MEDIUMS**
- ❏ 99mmTC
- ❏ 99mmTcDTPA
- ❏ Abrodil
- ❏ Acetiodone
- ❏ Acetrizoate
- ❏ Acetrizoic acid
- ❏ Albumotrope
- ❏ Aldosterone
- ❏ AN-DTPA Kit
- ❏ Angio-Conray
- ❏ Angiopac
- ❏ Angiotensin
- ❏ Apcitide
- ❏ Areteray
- ❏ Arteriodone
- ❏ Baridol
- ❏ Bariform
- ❏ barium sulfate
- ❏ Barosperse
- ❏ Barotrast
- ❏ BAS 16
- ❏ Bilgrafin
- ❏ Biliodyl
- ❏ Bilitrast
- ❏ Bilopaque
- ❏ Biloptin
- ❏ Bilospect
- ❏ bismuth carbonate
- ❏ calcium ipodate
- ❏ Campiodol
- ❏ CardioGen 82
- ❏ Cardiografin
- ❏ CardioTec Kit
- ❏ Cardiotrast
- ❏ CEA-SCAN
- ❏ Cesium 137
- ❏ chloriodized oil
- ❏ cholebrine
- ❏ Cholepelvis

- ❏ Choleradiagnostic
- ❏ Cholestim
- ❏ Cholevic
- ❏ Cholografin
- ❏ chromalbin
- ❏ chromic phosphate
- ❏ chromitope sodium
- ❏ Cis-Pyro Kit
- ❏ cobalt
- ❏ colloidal barium sulfate
- ❏ Conray
- ❏ cortisol
- ❏ Cysto-Conray
- ❏ deoxycorticosterone
- ❏ Diaginol
- ❏ Diagnorenol
- ❏ Diatrast
- ❏ diatrizoate
- ❏ digitoxin
- ❏ digoxin T-125
- ❏ Dimer-X
- ❏ Diodrast
- ❏ Dionosil
- ❏ diphosphonate
- ❏ disodium etidronate
- ❏ esriol
- ❏ Esophotrast
- ❏ ethiodized oil
- ❏ Ethiodol
- ❏ ferumoxide
- ❏ fluorescein
- ❏ gadiodiamide
- ❏ gallium citrate
- ❏ Gastrografin
- ❏ GastroMark
- ❏ Glofil-125
- ❏ Gold AU 198
- ❏ HD-85
- ❏ Hexabrix
- ❏ Hippuran I 131
- ❏ Hipputope

| ■ | X |
|---|---|

- ☐ hyaluronidase
- ☐ Hylenex
- ☐ Hytone
- ☐ Hypaque
- ☐ Hyskon
- ☐ Hytrast
- ☐ IC_Green
- ☐ Indium
- ☐ indocyanine green
- ☐ Iocetamic acid
- ☐ Iohexol
- ☐ iophendylate
- ☐ iothalamate
- ☐ ipodate
- ☐ Isopaque
- ☐ Lipiodol
- ☐ MDP kit
- ☐ meglumine
- ☐ methylglucamine
- ☐ metrizamide
- ☐ MMA kit
- ☐ MPI Iodine
- ☐ Myoview
- ☐ NeoTect
- ☐ Omnipaque
- ☐ Omniscan
- ☐ Oragrafin
- ☐ Oratrast
- ☐ OsteoScan
- ☐ Perchloracap
- ☐ pertechnetate sodium
- ☐ Phosphocol
- ☐ progesterone RIA
- ☐ propyliodone
- ☐ Quantisorb
- ☐ Renografin
- ☐ Reno-M-30
- ☐ Renotec
- ☐ Renovist
- ☐ Rubratope
- ☐ Salpix

| ■ | X |
|---|---|

- ☐ selenomethionine
- ☐ Sensor
- ☐ Sinaografin
- ☐ sodium chromate
- ☐ sodium diatrizoate
- ☐ sodium diphosphate
- ☐ sodium iodide
- ☐ sodium iodohippurate
- ☐ sodium pertechnetate
- ☐ sodium phosphate
- ☐ sodium rose Bengal
- ☐ sodium tyropanoate
- ☐ Strontium
- ☐ Technescan
- ☐ Technetium
- ☐ Telepaque
- ☐ Tensilon
- ☐ Tetrasorb
- ☐ Thyrolute
- ☐ Thyrostat
- ☐ Thyrotropin Alfa
- ☐ tricarbocyanine
- ☐ triolein
- ☐ Triosorb
- ☐ Vascoray
- ☐ Visipaque
- ☐ Xenon
- ☐ XE 133

www.ingramcontent.com/pod-product-compliance
Lightning Source LLC
Chambersburg PA
CBHW081126170526
45165CB00008B/2565

9 781439 226216